"Dr. Saic
trustworthy
to jump into
fully surrend
know it as the evolutionary force of love that it is."

Lisa Schrader, Founder, AwakeningShakti.com

"Desire is a must read for any person invested in living a fulfilling life while becoming at home with the powerful, guiding force of yearning."

Sage Lavine, #1 Best Selling Author: Women Rocking Business

"Saida takes us on a journey exploring all facets of desire - and how we each align with our life's calling to step into true sovereignty. It is a message of empowerment that all women should heed. The importance of connecting with pleasure in all the ways it shows up is critically important to quality of life and the key to activating the "switched-on life". Western Medicine has disconnected from extolling the importance of this pleasure connection for much of the past century. This book inspires me to commit to helping my patients prioritize pleasure and fully meet "desire" in their lives and relationships."

Debra Wickman, MD, FACOG

"This new creation, Desire, is a gorgeous read, an intimate journey into finding your own natural desire, that will bless you with tools to find the life you are yearning for, and the one that you deserve. Dr. Saida is a consummate guide to finding the wildness within ourselves, and the pleasure and comfort of our deep desire."

Dr. Rachel Carlton Abrams, MD, MHS, ABIM, Integrative Physician and Author of BodyWise: Discovering Your Body's Intelligence for Lifelong Health and Healing

"Dr. Saida Desilets is the most compelling and trustworthy guide that I have met to the deep wellspring of our human desire. She understands the daemon of desire, the prime directive in all its light and shadows, like few people teaching today. In her book, Desire, she offers with deep wisdom, achingly honest stories, and beautiful prose her learnings from a lifetime of exploring this profound, necessary, and shunned part of our lives, without which none of us can hope to find lasting joy or passion."

Doug Abrams, Co-Author of The Book of Joy

"It should be mandatory for every woman to read this book: your desires are crucial for evolution herself. Dare desire. Start your journey with desiring to devour this delicious book."

Kirsten Stendevad, Author of The Future is Feminine, www.kirstenstendevad.com

"What we deny and misunderstand holds the key to our greatest awakening. Dr. Saida Désilets leads us to reconciling our deepest yearning with our Soul's purpose: they are one and the same. Living this imbues our lives in grace."

Miranda Macpherson, Author of Boundless Love & The Way of Grace: the Transforming Power of Ego Relaxation

"Saida Desilets is a powerful force in the understanding of both the subtle and the apparent movement of DESIRE in any form. Fulfillment is everyone's birthright, and so I turn to Saida for many ways to achieve the satisfaction of a fulfilling life"

Caroline Muir, Author: Tantra Goddess

"Don't be fooled by this little book, it's a powerhouse of inspiration, daring, and clear paradigm shifts with regards to our relationship with desire, fulfillment and what it means to create a life we love."

Tanya Lynn, Author, Open Your Heart: How to be a New Generation Feminine Leader

"Dr. Saida Désilets reveals new facets of desire not yet considered, facets that not only are exhilarating to learn about, but also essential to designing and living our life in the ways we most dream of."

Elayne Kalila Doughty, Founder & Gatekeeper Priestess Presence

"This book is a graceful and delicious invitation to delve into the true power of desire. Saida takes you on a journey of awakening that dares you to take action to transform your life."

Rev. Monica Douglas-Clark, Spiritual Counsellor, and Author of The Reap Abundance Guidebook.

"Dr. Saida Desilets has set the new standard for how Leadership can transform the World in her new book Desire. Understanding and mastering our desire, channeling it for the benefit of many, we become more embodied, effective change makers without compromising what truly matters to us. A must read for all change makers."

Mitch Russo
Author of The Invisible Organization

"Saida has created far more than a book... It's a total Soul Ignition that shakes up and awakens all parts of you that has left enlightened Desire outside alone in the dark. Her wild tales captivate the heart and bring you to heal the fears and disbelief that you can actually have profound multidimensional Desire for yourself. Her approachable wisdom, coming from lifetimes of dedicated study and practice, will enter you, enlivening the gateways of your own ecstatic freedom and pleasure. Don't just read this... devour it fully to soar into realms of pleasure and love you can only imagine."

Satyen Raja
Founder of WarriorSage Trainings

"Saida's work is utterly life changing. For any woman that wants to know the magnitude of her power, brilliance and the deep intelligence that lives at the core of her heart and desires, I absolutely recommend you read this book!!!"

KC Baker, Founder and
CEO of WomanSpeak, Inc

"When we think of desire, we think of something personal -- something we want, something we need. But there's a level of desire that's much more fundamental — a desire that has nothing to do with who we think we are, and everything to do with who we really are. The real desire, is a fundamental yearning for oneness — a merging with the soul of humanity. In her newest book, Desire, Dr. Saida Desilets describes the essential journey of life, as a desire to, once again, fuse with the formless — the soul of life, the womb of creation. And, as we merge with the source, we disappear as an individual, and an awakening occurs to what has always been and what will always be — an awakening to our essence. Home at last!"

Jacob Israel Liberman, OD, PhD
Author of Luminous Life: How The Science Of
Light Unlocks The Art Of Living

Desire

By

Dr. Saida Désilets

Motivational Press
LEADERS IN GLOBAL PUBLISHING

Published by Motivational Press, Inc.
1777 Aurora Road
Melbourne, Florida, 32935
www.MotivationalPress.com

Photo by Caroline White Photography,
www.carolinewhitephotography.com

Manufactured in the United States of America.

ISBN: 978-1-62865-532-2

Contents

Ariel & Warwick ♡

May Desire's call be always heard & heeded… & may

To the spirit of Desire whom,
against all odds, still persistently
calls out to each of us, forever
dedicated to our enlivenment.

your hearts continually blossom ♡ Thank you for all your love & support ♡

[illegible] "hoMeMade" xoxo

Foreword by Tim Freke

I first met Saida in paradise. I'd been invited to speak in Maui and Saida, who was part of the team putting on the event, had been tasked with looking after me. From the moment we connected I knew I was in the presence of someone showing me, by example, a different way of being in the world.

I had never come across anyone so embodied and sensually alive. Here was someone at ease with pleasure, yet with clear, conscious boundaries. I felt I was encountering something wild and untamed. Yet I also felt nurtured by someone kind and encouraging, with a sophisticated understanding of the human condition.

So I was honoured when Saida asked me to write a foreword for this daring book about 'desire', because I want to support her expressing in words the wisdom she embodies.

Desire and Spirituality

Desire is the power that propels life forward. Our passions urge us to realise new possibilities. What we want we strive to create. Yet most traditional forms of spirituality have taken a dim view of desire. We're told it binds us to a world we need to escape. It disturbs our equanimity. It leads to suffering.

This traditional perceptive is based on the idea of the 'Fall'. We are souls who have been cast out of some better place and need to get home. We are God who has become lost in His own dream. We are captives caught in an illusion from which we need to liberate ourselves.

What keeps us prisoners in the world is our human nature. Most of the characteristics that define our humanity are bad and must be eradicated. Thinking is bad. Emotional attachments are bad. Desires are really bad ... particularly lust which is utterly deplorable. Having spent my life studying, experiencing and writing about world spirituality, I am convinced we need to replace the pessimistic philosophy of the 'Fall' with the optimistic idea of 'Evolution', which underlies modern science.

The whole universe is evolving and through this creative process new qualities of existence continually emerge into being. Existence is always evolving into something greater. You and I are evolving and can continually realise more of our potential.

So, it seems to me, we need to create a new 'emergent' form of spirituality that still guides us to the transcendent, as our ancient traditions do, but also encourages us to consciously engage with the evolutionary adventure.

We need a positive spirituality that inspires us to embrace the bittersweet journey of life. A human-centred spiritually that urges to be embodied ... to feel and think ... to desire and dare.

Passive and Active Love

The central insight that has arisen for me from my experience of spiritual awakening is that the most important thing in life is love. And love has a passive and an active aspect, which complement each other perfectly.

Passive love arises when we become conscious of the stillness of our Deep Being, from which we can unconditionally accept and appreciate the moment just as it is. Active love arises as the passionate desire to make things better, for ourselves and each other.

In my book Deep Awake while exploring 'love' and 'desire', I wrote the following, which I feel just as strongly today ...

"I would hate to become a passionless person. I want to feel a fire burning in my belly. A yearning to live and express myself. A longing for a better world. I don't just want to feel at peace with life as it is. I also want to experience the tempestuous rush of new possibilities struggling within me to be born. I want to feel the heat of desire. The urgent pangs of hunger for more. The defiant will to grow."

Desire isn't bad, it can be beautiful, righteous, even holy. But desire isn't necessarily good either, because it's what we desire that counts. If our desires focus only on personal benefit and animal needs, they will limit and confine us. But if we awaken our most emergent desires, we will find ourselves in service to the greatest good.

If we can hear the call of a better future ... if we feel the need to respond to the evolutionary impulse that propels us forward ... then, as Saida urges us in this book, we must uncover our deepest desires and be daring enough to follow where they lead.

Some years ago I met another powerful woman who inspired me. This lady was in her eighties and we connected briefly as strangers for a spontaneous conversation in a coffee bar. As I prepared to leave, having shared how much I had enjoyed our meeting, I squeezed her hand and said sweetly 'Take care'. The lady looked me in the eyes and replied in a voice full of age and wisdom ... 'No. Take a risk!'

Tim Freke

Deep Awake Philosopher, Author of Soul Story

Foreword by Dr. Lissa Rankin

Desire. How easily it confuses us! To live a deeply fulfilling life, are we meant to follow the teachings of dominant culture, which encourage us to "Just do it," grasping for our desires, using will and force to "make it happen?" Or are we supposed to visualize, affirm, meditate, and create vision boards about what we desire so we can leverage our spiritual power to "manifest" our wishes? Are we better off surrendering our desires to some Higher Power, leaving only the desire to align with Divine Will? Are we meant to lean into our desire as Rumi and the Sufis do—reveling in the deliciousness of unmet longing as a path to that which we ultimately desire—the Beloved?

According to this book, the answer would "Yes. And Yes. And Yes. And Hell Yeah!"

In both worldly and spiritual traditions, desire can leave us with our panties in a wad of bewilderment, yet, perhaps if we can handle the discomfort of holding infinite paradoxes, we can feel the unbearably pleasurable experience of leaning all the way into our desires while simultaneously trusting a mysterious force of love that participates in the co-creation of our desires- and also dismantles them.

Whether we like it or not, desire is a force to be reckoned with by us mortal Divine humans. To suggest that it's even possible to be some desire-less zombie can be misleading and befuddling. But even if it were possible, why would we want to disconnect ourselves from the sweet nectar of our juiciest longings? After all, every creation begins as a desire- every baby born into the world, every story that becomes a book, every kiss that becomes a partnership, every sculpture that emerges from the marble's desire to become something beautiful and the artist's desire to participate with this creative impulse. This oh-so-human "daemonic" impulse (not to be confused with the "demonic") carries within it both the life force and the death force. If we suppress the life force inherent in healthy desire, it comes out sideways, either in its fiery forms of violence, rage, and abuses of power, or in its life force-dimming loss of vitality via depression, anxiety, chronic illness, decreased libido, addiction, and suicidal ideation.

Yet grasping for everything we desire doesn't seem to create lasting fulfillment either. Expending all of your energy trying to fill some "hungry ghost" hole inside rarely works. No amount of sex, money, fame, achievement, or hedonistic pleasure fulfills us for long. In *The How Of Happiness,* professor Sonja Lyubomirsky, PhD shares the data about what makes us more happy- and what doesn't. It turns out that, because of "hedonistic adaptation," only 10% of our happiness depends on the fulfillment of our desires. In other words, even if you get everything you think you want, your happiness will only improve a small amount. Although you may feel happier temporarily, very quickly, this effect wears off, and you're likely to start grasping for the next shiny, sparkly thing.

So what is a yearning, longing, deliciously hungry being supposed to do with all this human longing? Distancing yourself from your desires doesn't seem to work either. Pretending to be non-attached and numbing your deepest desires fools nobody, especially not your precious, wanting human heart. This spiritual bypassing tool may make you feel less vulnerable, but really this pain-avoidance technique of pretending you don't want what you want only leaves the vulnerable, longing part feeling exiled. You may feel like you hurt less if you pretend you don't have desires, but deep down, the exiled longing part is a hurting thing, just craving your love, affection, and acknowledgment.

Like it or not, to be human is to want.

The Buddha suggests that all suffering arises from the attachment to the desire to get what we want and avoid what we don't want, but what if we don't need to run away from suffering? What if it's the running away from suffering that saps our life force? What if these natural human cravings and aversions are a vital part of the human experience, and pain is an alchemical crucible inviting us into a deeper, richer life, something we don't need to avoid, something we could actually lean into- with gratitude, even- if only we dared.

Love warrior Glennon Doyle Melton teaches that we run away from our desires because if we actually stay in the fire of them, we have to feel the "hot loneliness" that accompanies unrealized desires. Because we don't like feeling the hot loneliness, we have a tendency to look for "Easy buttons" that can help us avoid feeling it. But what if the hot loneliness is not something to run away from either?

Glennon writes, "Everything we need to become the people we were meant to become next is actually inside the hot loneliness of now. So when we Easy button our way out, we are like caterpillars who jump out of the cocoon right before we would have become butterflies. Because pain is actually not a hot potato. It's the traveling professor, and it knocks on everybody's door. The wisest ones say, 'Come in. Sit down, and don't leave until you've taught me what I need to know.' But we've got it all wrong. We are afraid of pain, but we were made for pain. We need to be afraid of the Easy buttons. Because the journey of the Love Warrior is to rush toward her pain and let her pain become her power.

What if our desires- whether realized or not- can become a tool for transformation? What if what we most want actually lives inside the ecstasy and the agony of our most vulnerable longings? Mystics express that our deepest desire is to experience our own wholeness, to feel our Oneness with all things, to dive into the rapture of simply being alive, and to fall in love with and unite with the Divine Beloved inside our own hearts. Yet, as humans, we all bear the Original Wound of separation. We were once part of the collective ocean, and then by splitting off our consciousness as a drop of the ocean and incarnating in a body, we feel an almost unbearable longing to be part of the ocean again.

We may be blessed to experience the fulfillment of this desire for Oneness in moments of ecstasy- during rapturous sex or deep meditation or expanded consciousness out in nature or while using plant medicines. Yet such experiences of mystical union are usually temporary, wearing off as the story of separation takes hold again, leaving us with the agonizing memory of how fulfilling it feels to be the ocean and how sad, lonely, and despairing it can feel when we are a separate drop!

So what is a healthy human daemon to do? Dare we chase after all the fickle desires that capture our attention? Or are we better off ignoring all those shiny, sparkly distractions? How can we handle the many songs of desire that sing in our hearts, longing for expression and fulfillment? Dare we allow ourselves the vulnerability of actually feeling our deepest unmet longings all the way?

Within the pages you're about to read lie many wise answers, often cloaked in the paradoxes that reveal the deep wisdom and juicy, embodied aliveness of the one who has written them. This book will take you on one of the longest pilgrimages you'll ever take- that sometimes arduous but hopefully delicious journey from the head to the heart- and in this case, the gut, and- if you're lucky- the pelvis. Trust Saida to help you navigate this sometimes confusing terrain. The very feminine maps she offers will not promise where you'll end up, but you're guaranteed to enjoy the ride.

Lissa Rankin, MD

New York Times bestselling author of
Mind Over Medicine, The Fear Cure,
The Anatomy of a Calling, and
What's Up Down There?

Desire is my voice.

I'm the translator between realms.

I speak through desire.

Desire is not a thing she's a being.

She's the Daemon of our aliveness.

She's the achingly beautiful song that breaks our icy rigidity and dispels the practical. Yet she's the most practical.

We are not meant to be machines, we are meant to express life in all our moments.

Life is doing us. Breathing us. Living us. Leading us, yet so few of us are truly alive.

Note to the Reader

All the stories shared in this book are true stories, retold with as much accuracy as possible. However, when names are used, they have been changed to protect the privacy of the mentioned individual(s). Some of the stories may appear to be fantastical, yet every description is as true and real as you breathing right now while reading these words.

READER RESOURCES

Companion Playbook

Do you love applying ideas to your own life? We've created a companion Desire Playbook filled with questions exploring the ideas from each chapter. It's free and available for instant download at: **DesireTheBook.Club**

Companion Videos:

Throughout this book you'll come upon this symbol:

When it shows up, it indicates that there's a companion video explaining this part of the book more thoroughly. These are recorded discussions between Dr. Saida & her community. They are free and available instantly at: **DesireTheBook.Club**

Why Desire, Why Now?

Desire is an emergent, evolutionary and ambivalent force.

It can lead us into experiencing profound fulfillment or leave us depleted, worn out, jaded, and no closer to fulfillment than when we first began our earnest striving, ticking all the boxes off our socially mandated to-do list.

Yet, beneath our entire bustle, frustration, and numbing habits, lives our true desire, silently whispering to us, calling us back home to ourselves.

Existing in a predetermined world that has all but eradicated the wonder from our hearts, feels like being busy getting nowhere fast. Yet still, even there, in the midst of our sleepless nights, our own desire pulses, awaiting the one moment when we may finally whisper: *I dare...*

Living a daring life isn't just about jumping off cliffs and asking a random stranger on a date. Living a daring life includes, being willing to get out of bed when it's the last thing we feel like doing.

A daring life is dedicated to listening to, taking pleasure in, and following without compromise the visceral sensation of our soul's calling—a song of desire that is exhilarating, liberating, and uniquely our own.

I believe we each possess a prime directive, a life-current that is purely ours, and that it's our greatest act in this life to realize and to shamelessly express this true version of ourselves.

Coming Home to Ourselves

Death smiled in my face on three separate occasions. Perhaps this alone has given me a unique understanding that life is incredibly precious and delicate, and we must live as though today is truly our last.

It's possible that my violent, near-death rape experience and my ensuing journey of recovery, ignited within me my true calling—a devotion to reminding women of their greatness, calling them back home to themselves so they too could remember their own sovereign space (their body) and shamelessly claim and express their version of femininity.

In recent years, I've noticed a fierce compassion emerging from within me, influencing how I lead and facilitate, resulting in a change with my language, where the word *daring* has taken dominance. Daring is part of every woman's choice to move toward something she innately feels is possible, despite the lack of evidence of its expression in her world.

I witness an act of extreme daring whenever a woman finally chooses to love her body the way it is, especially in the face of all the social pressures to have the perfect ageless, perky, receptive, orgasmic body.

I notice it's exceptionally daring for a woman to surrender to her own pleasure, because to do so is an act of defiance against the social pressures. To be the perfect woman who sacrifices all for others, who can be a perfect mother while running a perfect and successful business, and maintaining an uber-sexy and fulfilling, perfect relationship.

Every day I see daring in action when a woman finally admits to herself the inner yearnings of her heart, while also knowing her current situation is nowhere close to reflecting this vision.

It takes daring to be willing to be a messy human. Yet, messy humans are the only real humans.

The rest are just a world of zombies, infected by rote ideals and social conformity.

Ironically, even those who believe they are sexually liberated and free, are often acting out a mandate demanded by social norms.

And yet, when my desire is my true north and I'm willing to dare into whatever emerges in the choice to express this desire, I notice something exquisite happens: I suddenly experience genuine fulfillment—not as a fleeting sensation, but as a bone-deep truth that permeates all my moments. I'm filled with a deep sense of purpose, of belonging, a feeling that my life matters, and that what I create is a worthy contribution.

The Beauty of Daring Into Our Desires

For as long as I can remember, I've had a finger, sometimes literally, on the pulse of my desire. Yes, at times I've experienced the pain and heartbreak of pursuing hijacked desires—

socially mandated desires that we mistake as our own—however, even then, beneath this experience, was the undeniable pulse of my soul.

What's gorgeous about this daring way of living is there's never a dull moment. We are in a constant, ever-creative, emerging relationship with life itself, meeting that which is already moving toward us, with a sense of openness, adventure, and wonderment.

I'm profoundly privileged to champion women's sexual sovereignty, inviting them into the simple, yet challenging journey back home to themselves.

This is true no matter her age, size, ethnicity, income level, education, social status, marital status, and so forth. Because more than all her other socially mandated roles, a woman is a unique current of femininity, and when she comes home to this living truth, she becomes the force of nature she was born to be.

That is a breathtaking and worthy cause.

Perhaps one of the greatest atrocities of our time is the disruption of a person's inborn sovereignty. It's my firm belief that no person, governing body, or religious state has the right to depict what happens to our sovereign space—our body. Our body is sacred, it's the vehicle through which we experience life and from which our most essential contributions flow.

It's through our body that we sense the physicality of our desire's calling. We experience this as an undeniable yearning, one so strong we are compelled to act. Perhaps this is why religions and governments of old, made it their sanction to regulate, restrict, and rationalize desire so they, and we, have some semblance of control when it comes to this powerful human force.

Yet, this suppression has not created a better world. Instead, it has led us to where we find ourselves today: our body and our sexuality are commodities that appear to lose more value the further along we are in our preordained life. The life designed to make us a good, healthy, and appropriate citizen of the world.

Daring into our true desires, isn't just for the promise of better sex, love, parenting, fulfillment, contribution, and devotional rapture—it's for us to hear and heed the prime directive that lives within each of us.

Humans and domesticated animals are the only beings who get confused about their place in the world. Yet, through this single act of shifting from the pervasive influence of social directives into choosing a creative orientation to our own life, we unfetter our natural abilities. We begin using our inborn compass, moving toward our own true north, daring to take a step, no matter how big or small, toward the YES of living our soul's true calling.

It is my wish to take you on a journey to meet a very vital part of yourself, your own daemon of desire. Think of your daemon as the translating spirit between yourself and the mystery we call life. She has the capacity to know the true nature of your own fulfillment; she has the songs that will call you into a direct, vibrant relationship with the ever-emerging story that is your unique life.

I invite you to dare, dare into everything you've ever deeply (and secretly) yearned for, to breathe life into this part of yourself, and to allow a spaciousness to exist wherein all that you are as a complete (and messy) human is invited to have a profoundly intimate relationship with life itself.

Prologue

"I do not at all understand the mystery of grace—only that it meets us where we are, but does not leave us where it found us."

Anne Lamott

July 1999, Russell Island, Canada

Blindfolded, we're running full tilt, straining to keep up with the sounds of the shaman's feet up ahead. For the most part I stayed right behind him, but I stumbled into a few crevices, leaving part of my shin smeared along the sharp rock.

The worst moment was when I couldn't hear him running anymore. I realized, with a sudden twist in my stomach, that he'd jumped off a cliff, and I would have to surrender fully and follow suit.

Jumping blindfolded off a cliff is nothing short of terrifying, yet, when I abruptly landed just a few feet below, I burst out laughing at my unnecessary fear. Having passed some test, we were free to unveil our eyes and squint into the late-afternoon sun.

It was but a few moments later that the shaman asked me to lead an exercise to help everyone come back into their sensual body. Surprised, but honored, I knew exactly what to share.

The exercise was simple and very sensual. One partner would lie on their front, while the other sat on their back, with their sitting-bones on either side of the spine of the receiving partner. The giver moved slowly in undulating circles, slowly making their way up from the receiver's butt to the receiver's shoulder blades and then back down again.

A deep sadness infected me—perhaps emerging from the sense of separation from the group since I was leading and could not partake in the intimate experience. Even more bizarre, I simultaneously noticed a strong, persistent heartbeat in my perineum. I assumed, at first, it was my own rhythmic heart, but when I checked my own pulse, they clearly were mismatched.

That's when a tangible weirdness started to grow. The deep rumble of an emerging storm front, mixing with a sudden rise in the wind and the loud screeching of a circling bald eagle..."Stop!" The Shaman suddenly rose and cried out, "Someone is channeling something powerful. Who is it? Please come forward."

Immensely curious, due to the rising sound of my own experience, I also exclaimed, "Yeah, please show yourself!"

No one moved.

Even though the energy of the brewing storm was boiling over to the point of intolerable intensity. Again, the Shaman cried out, "This is very powerful. Please come forward. Do not be afraid. Please speak up."

Again, I agreed and exclaimed, "Yes! Speak up!!" As I looked through the group, wondering who was stirring such intensity, everyone appeared passive, unmoved.

Then, out of the blue, a surge of enormous intensity burst through the bottoms of my feet and sizzled through my entire body, leaving me stunned and yelling. Imagine the best orgasm you've ever had, combined with a thousand volts of energy. Stunned from the electrifying sensation, I took a deep breath in.

That's when a second surge came through, only this time it was equivalent to ten thousand volts. I literally had to scream as the painful, yet ecstatic, electric current illuminated my entire body so completely that I involuntarily arched backward.

When it was over, I was left panting and bewildered. However, before I could even try to understand what was happening, a third wave of now one hundred thousand volts of ecstatic electricity, rushed up from the earth, penetrating every fiber of my body. This left me screaming with unbridled intensity, while arching so fully backward that my head was only inches from the ground.

Finally, when I was released, I found myself standing, stunned, and looking into the confused eyes of the Shaman. "Stop, you must stop this now! You are terrifying everyone."

I looked around to find the support of my tribe, but they uncomfortably averted their eyes, unable to process the inexplicable phenomenon they had just been witness to. I turned back to the Shaman for support, but instead received a disapproving scowl. At this, I burst into tears as I fell to the ground, feeling more alien than human.

I wasn't on any drugs or medicinal plants and I certainly wasn't drunk or altered in any way. This all occurred unintentionally, without ritual or ceremony. It scared the living crap out of everyone—including the one we all counted on for steadfastness and wisdom.

Then, suddenly everyone around me started having sex. We are on a spiritual vision quest, not a wild sex camp where orgies would make sense.

The sight and sound of crude human sex, felt exceptionally awful to my newly Earth-ravaged awareness. It felt like they were attempting, but failing miserably, to replicate the exalted current I had just been penetrated by.

Unable to handle another second of this lowly grasping, I ran off, blinded by tears, into the deep dark of the forest. I spent the entire night curled up in the fetal position, alternating between calm and stillness, paranoia and fear. A swarm of mosquitoes came and went with my wavering consciousness like an undulating blanket. This battle went on for most of the night, until I somehow managed to collapse into oblivion.

When I woke, it was as though I was seeing the world for the first time. The rainbow sun rays, pouring through the green of the massive cedars, the softness of the earth beneath me, and the sweet chirping of the forest life.

The beauty of being alive cracked me open and unbridled love and bliss filled me until I experienced myself at one with everything around me, as if I was making love with life itself.

A crew of playful hummingbirds swooped in around me as though I was a living, walking blossom, accompanying me back to camp. It was as though they wanted to remind me I had not dreamt any of this, that it was as real as the reliable rising of the sun.

CHAPTER 1

THE DEMONIC SIDE OF DESIRE

Few are those who see with their own eyes
and feel with their own hearts.
Albert Einstein

It wasn't always like this.

There was a time when we followed our desires and were either rewarded for the exploration or died in the attempt—ingesting poisonous plants, entering croc invested waters, dying of dehydration through journeying into unknown territory. Either way, we could not resist desire even if we wanted to. It was our primal compass.

In my young heart, I felt there was some sort of inexplicable magic behind the veil of our mundane existence. This orientation helped me digest the atrocities that inundated both my own private life and the world at large.

That moment on Russell Island changed me forever. I could no longer ignore that something much greater was at stake, something no one else seemed to be aware of or care about. I yearned to understand why I had been chosen and how that sort of power could even exist, let alone affect me physically.

So I devoted myself to the study of sensuality and deep orgasm. I would come to find out there were just as much dogma and entrapment in the so-called "spiritual-sexual" pursuit, as there was in "normal, mainstream" life.

"To teach you the advanced activation formula, we'll need to perform the rite of sacred, sexual union. I'll activate within you your energy centers and you will know bliss beyond anything you've ever known." This was the promise contained in the email from my current guide in the arts of Taoist sexuality.

I was intrigued, I wanted all the powers and promises of this ancient practice: eternal youth, immortality, and knowing God through sex.

Therefore, we met, in the attic bedroom of my best friend's house. He was her boyfriend, but somehow he didn't think what we were about to do was a betrayal. I went along with his guidance since he was thirty-four years older than me.

We performed the sacred rite—but for me it was just sex, and not even great sex at that. There was no sensuality, no foreplay, and he couldn't even sustain a strong erection. The most fascinating part was the contorted athletic position, which was at least new and exotic.

I was open and willing and dutifully waited for the "big bang," for God to show himself, for my world to be shattered by the immortal blessing from this ancient rite. What I was met with was more like: *Meh.*

Nothing happened except for lame sex.

He acted like it was the most extraordinary blessing, while I felt empty inside.

When our desires are based on the values and ideals that others have impressed upon us, we are playing with the demonic side of desire. Learned desire, or hijacked desire, falls short of delivering true fulfillment, and that is simply because it cannot. Only true desire that emerges from the depth of our own inherent knowing, can possibly offer us fulfillment.

I understand now, after many years of walking this Earth—part-human and part-daemon—that human life is exceptionally messy and modern living is excruciatingly demanding. I've seen how easy it is to find ourselves at the mercy of a million different desires, most of which seem to have come out of nowhere. We exhaust ourselves in an attempt to fulfill each and every one of them.

We are unique individuals, having our own experiences and creating from our own version of reality. Yet, we spend most of our time attempting to fit into some cookie-cutter version of what we are supposed-to-be-so-we-can-belong. How long can we keep up without falling prey to depression and exhaustion?

Our ancient human need to survive through belonging has become a detriment to our very survival.

"The young always have the same problem—
how to rebel and conform at the same time.
They have now solved this by defying their
parents and copying one another."

Quentin Crisp

It's our uniqueness, rather than our ability to blend in, that leads to creating a fulfilling life within ourselves. But in a society where uniqueness is dictated by trending cultural memes, we end up operating under the guise of independence, while we're really just slaves to conformity.

So what is leading us to numb ourselves out with social media, drugs, alcohol, or sex—or even attempting to take our own lives?

Desire.

Not the true nature of our desire, but the trickster version of desire.

We are inundated from pre-birth, and throughout our life, with strong social constructs, which instill in us an unspoken map of how we should or shouldn't live our lives.

For most of us, this formula spells disaster.

Even if we somehow manage to juggle all these predetermined ideals, we end up burning ourselves out in the attempt to maintain the status quo.

Desire's call cannot go unheard. It's an achingly poignant siren call within all of us: keeping us up at night, throbbing within us during the rote routines of our life, constantly vying for our attention.

Desire is both personal and impersonal, it's inborn within each of us, as it's inborn within all of life. However, because of her ambivalent nature, desire cares not how we use her arousing call—she only cares that we heed it.

Which is why desire can appear demonic. Whether we act unconsciously or with the semblance of consciousness, when we are following the call of hijacked desires, we will never experience true fulfillment—and worse, we'll be stripped of the very life we yearn to ignite.

"In the USA alone, on average, there are 121 suicides and 3,025 suicide attempts per day. That's over 1,104,125 attempts per year."

American Foundation for Suicide Prevention

Suicide isn't just a consideration for the desperate; it's the act we all undertake when we are not living in alignment with our own true north, the essential calling of our Desire.

How do we face the insurmountable pressures of social conformity? How can we ever truly know if we are enacting our true Desires or subject to the lure of hijacked desires? And what's the point of even attempting to understand?

Our life depends upon our capacity to hear and heed the true voice of our desire.

Chapter 2

The Symphony of Desire

You call God's greatest gift—ourselves, our yearning, our need to love—you call it filth and sin and heresy...

Veronica Franco, Dangerous Beauty

I lie on the floor of my apartment, face down in a pool of tears. Everything I had ever desired in my dream relationship was shattered with finality: him hanging up the phone.

He was the one who insisted we get married right away. To me, it had the "smell of God." I went along with it just to see what would emerge from this outrageous request.

I remember the day I attempted to fly to him, but the airplane never took off. For eight hours we sat at the gate and for eight hours I denied the deep voice inside of me that kept saying, "This relationship will never take off..."

And it didn't.

One month after the wedding, he asked me, over the phone, to annul the marriage.

Yet for me, I'd said the words, "forever and ever." Surely forever was longer than thirty-two days?

I stopped eating for three months—looking like a heroine junkie, yet receiving compliments from women about how "hot" I looked. This struck me as sinister, since inside I felt withered, on a fast path to a sure death.

Luckily for me, that morning on the floor, I was finally brave enough to open my eyes and peer at the monster living within my darkest depths. I gasped at what I saw: only pure love looking back.

Our relationship to our desires are a clear reflection of how we relate to all of life. For the most part, we are both fascinated and terrified of the power of our desires.

Left to freely explore our desire for ourselves, we may eventually come to realize the truth about our desire. However, there's an unseen, yet all-pervasive, roadblock to the free exploration of this inborn human quality: *the mass hypnosis and universal influence of consumerism, social conditioning, and domestication.*

This ever-consensual, social tendency polarizes our experience of desire. We are either influenced to fully indulge in every tiny desire the second it arises or shut down and numb out so that we do not have to feel the mystery that lies on the edge of our yearning.

To add fuel to this fire, the consistent entrapment of our own beliefs about desire misleads us, until we're like the walking dead, rather than enlivened humans.

Equally troubling is we seem to enjoy perpetuating this zombie-like virus, eagerly willing to infect one another with our conditioned truths about desire. Unfortunately, the more innocent a person is—the more free, open, and present—the more eager we are to infect them.

Like young children.

Children are the gatekeepers of life and as such, we should treat them with profound reverence, seek their council and join them in meaningless, unproductive play.

Instead, our cultural mandate, ensures they are properly socialized for the good of their survival. We've all experienced this as children: no one escapes the process of domestication.

On one level, it's absolutely necessary. It ensures we understand the rules of conduct, language, and other social constructs that comprise living in peace with one another.

That being said, it's important to understand that buried well beneath the shiny surface, lives the truth of our own nature.

We are all born wealthy, our "bank accounts" are infinite, yet we believe we have nothing—and worse, that we need to fill this emptiness with something.

What is beautiful about our desire is it's the emerging treasure of our most essential nature. We all share in the common experience of yearning for what we don't have, and if we are courageous enough to follow and realize this impulse, we actually get to enjoy what emerges to meet us.

If it's love we yearn for, we'll move toward love. If it's a family we yearn for, we'll move toward creating a family and so forth.

Unfortunately, our conditioning teaches us to yearn for the experience of fulfillment as though it is a *promise* of fulfillment —something we will eventually have. This is the lie of our false desires because in actuality, our true desire is already innately fulfilled: we already are what we yearn for.

Fulfillment is a coming home to self. All true desires are simply an invitation into the realization that, our desires become viable through the arising of our yearning.

So the culprit in living a zombie-life, lies within our false or hijacked desires, since they have entrained us all to be numb and blind to fulfillment. To be a person who yearns for love, yet turns away from love everyday—behaving like a beggar, jealous of the love others have, or worse, acting as a thief, stealing and poisoning any existing love that shows up.

Resolving desire isn't the intention of our true desire.

Desire is a magnetic quality, intended to pull us toward what we already are. Desire isn't meant to be resolved: in fact, at times, its resolution can lead to feeling unfulfilled.

To experience true fulfillment, we must love our desire. Our desire is our soul's voice igniting, inspiring, and enlivening us. Bringing us into life, infusing us with the awareness that we belong to life, that this belonging isn't something that goes away.

Many of us have suffered through our primal need to belong. When we recognize that we already belong to life itself, in that moment we experience fulfillment.

Every one of us has a unique code, a prime directive, a raison d'être.

Every one of us runs a unique current, our own offering that is gifted to this life, purely for the sake of itself and that is true fulfillment.

They say there are moments in life that are poignant and we'll see them flash before our eyes when we die. This was one of those moments.

On one hand, there I was, quietly sitting in my mediation chair, surrounded by the quiet of my apartment and the fragrance of tuberose that I'd brought home that morning.

On the other hand, I was sitting on a warm rock in the hot Egyptian sun. The priest came for me and we walked in silence into the Great

Pyramid, where I knew my way into the king's chamber. It was my sole role to midwife the pharaoh into the other world. Royal blue and gold swirled from him as he left his earthly body behind.

I felt completely at home in this experience, as if I'd done it a multitude of times. And yet, as I took a full breath, I was just a young single woman, exploring the deeper arts of intentional meditation.

What fascinated me the most about this moment was that, later, my Egyptologist friend, confirmed that the path I took to get to the king's chamber, was indeed the actual existing path—down to the last detail!

How could I be in two places at once? How could I possibly know that place and that ceremony when I'd never physically set foot in Egypt or studied anything about Egyptians?

Unable to explain the living truth of my experience, but feeling remarkably nourished and fulfilled, I stored this experience in the place within me where the magical elements of my life reside.

If desire is the daemon linking us directly to our souls—the sensorial voice that draws us more fully into the realization of fulfillment—and fulfillment isn't the end goal, but a doorway into life itself, then what happens if our dominant experience of desire is denying it?

If we are terrified of actual fulfillment, what does that say about us?

For one, it says we never truly live. Rather, we consistently live through others, their joy, their success, their beauty, and their pain. Perhaps that's why billions of people worldwide are addicted to soap operas and social media.

But what if, for a moment, we could truly live for ourselves—what would that look like?

Desire shows up in unique ways, in the form of songs that belong to the symphony of life. Although, each song may appear to be unique and separate from the other songs, they are all actually an intricate part of this greater symphony.

Desire emerges through a variety of unique, yet interconnected songs: the Song of Eros, the Song of Rapture, the Song of Love, the Song of Procreation, the Song of Thriving, and the Song of Contribution.

True Desire doesn't care about how, when or whom it sings through—it only cares about being that consistent call bringing us back to ourselves.

Desire doesn't care about right or wrong, she just is.

Desire has always been part of this universe, how else would everything have come into existence if there weren't some sort of primordial force desiring to expand and know itself?

There was a moment, when I was two weeks shy of thirteen, when I experienced myself as clearly separate from my body.

The propane gas had leaked throughout the night, so with the strike of a match, our entire camper van blew up and I was thrown straight through the wall. Writhing in agony in the gravel, I was screaming and aching, yet somehow completely detached from what my body was experiencing.

In truth, I was actually sitting in a cozy chair looking out of the two big circular windows—the orbs of my eyes. Everything was tranquil, quiet, my body's agony wasn't felt, it was fascinating.

I observed my body pick itself up and run into the cold lake next to our campsite.

That's when I "came to," bewildered, wondering why I was sitting in the lake and what the heck the weird stuff hanging off my arms was.

As I started to pull on this strange webbing, I suddenly realized it was my skin; it melted off me so that it was hanging like thin silk from my arms. That's when I started to scream, all semblance of control was lost.

What remained was the question: If I'm not my body, who or what am I?

Desire has the capacity to bring forth something from nothing, for example, the miracle of conception. In one moment there is nothing—in the next there is the start of life!

This impulse is one of the prime directives of life and it exists outside of our social constructs, ideals, religious beliefs and political structures.

But desire is much more than just the miracle of procreation; it's our pure creative impulse.

Let's imagine the beginning of this universe—a primordial impulse to exist and know itself. We have the initial change of non-matter into matter.

Desire has both an evolutionary and an emerging quality to it: from the primordial, to the primal, to survival, to reproduction, and onward. As our survival blossomed, we blossomed, with each evolutionary step, a new form of desire emerged—ever unfolding, ever pulling us forward to explore, discover and create anew.

If we look at different points in our history, we can see shifts in our evolution as each new emerging calling was felt and expressed.

We are no different now.

Desire continues to emerge and to pull us forward into our next evolutionary expression. In this way, we can say desire is both the inspiration and the fuel to make that inspiration real.

Yet, desire is more than just a motivational, action-oriented force. It is quite literally the calling of our soul (or what the ancient Greeks referred to as our psyche) speaking through our physicality.

Desire is not only a mental construct—but equally, and more honestly, a visceral felt-sense throughout our body. We cannot deny its pull toward something that deeply inspires us, awakens us, and fuels us.

Which brings us back to the concept of fulfillment.

Fulfillment doesn't mean the end.

We are all terrified of the end, utterly incapacitated by the idea of dying. Therefore, we actually avoid true fulfillment because we fear if we have it, there will no longer be a purpose to our lives.

Fulfillment, true fulfillment, is dynamic because it is life in its full expression. Desire never stops—she evolves. She will always sing your heart song until the moment you die.

Fulfillment cares nothing of where we are born, to whom, in which country, or where we're headed. True fulfillment only cares about HOW ALIVE WE ARE RIGHT NOW!

"Do you know what you are? You are a manuscript of a divine letter. You are a mirror reflecting a noble face. This universe is not outside of you. Look inside yourself; everything that you want, you are already that."

Rumi

This is why it's a crime to go toward hijacked desires. However, it isn't our fault we do: we do because we don't know better, because we've been infected with the virus. This virus only has power against those of us who believe in it.

Desire doesn't require your belief.

Desire exists free from the confines of your mind: she is the daemon dancing life into you. And yes, hijacked desire is what most of us know: We are taught that in order to have fulfillment, we must have this or that, and we believe it. We cease to be alive until we have it—and yet when we finally do get it, we feel more dead inside.

In the resolution of false/hijacked desire, we kill ourselves. We become the living dead—numb, unable to feel, and therefore, perpetuating our global addiction to sensation. We are all addicts, and as addicts we can never feel satisfied, we always want more.

To become free, sovereign, truly alive human beings, we must recognize our dissatisfaction and let go of all our judgments about desire and consumerism. Otherwise, we continually perpetuate the polarity that domestication so neatly sets up.

"By overcoming the desire to satisfy, please, impress, or better others, we can start living for ourselves, free from unnatural and destructive desires."

Neel Burton

Desire is our birthright, it's desire that brings us into the world. It's desire that shimmers with our last breath because desire is life.

The purpose of our lives isn't fulfillment, we are born fulfilled. The purpose of our lives is to BE fulfilled. Whole. Radiant. As enlivened as life itself—dynamic, pure, raw, wild, vulnerable, soft, intense, and devastating.

Desire, true desire, awaits each of us, never lost, just patient. She expresses herself through a myriad of unique songs, never critical, just present. The second we turn our attention to our true desire is the moment we ignite ourselves and come into being fully here, fully home, and fully filled with life.

CHAPTER 3

THE DESIRE SONG OF EROS

"Civilization is a process in the service of Eros, whose purpose is to combine single human individuals, and after that families, then races, peoples and nations, into one great unity, the unity of mankind. Why this has to happen, we do not know; the work of Eros is precisely this."

Sigmund Freud

I love sex, I've loved it my entire life. I especially discovered how much I loved it the very first time I had sex with another person.

It was with a skateboarding gang member. I thought he was so hot, and bad enough to be interesting, yet sweet, because he knew my friend Tracy and she was the kindest person I knew.

We met at a club; I had Tracy tell him I wanted to fuck him, but not that night. I had her arrange that he and I talk and make plans: to meet on Friday night, at my house, while my family was away for the weekend.

I was just shy of turning eighteen and very sure that he was the one.

Thankfully, he was both skilled and conscious—he brought condoms.

What I wasn't prepared for was the size of him—I had no idea how he'd fit (but wow, did he ever fit!). The tingling I felt from toe to head afterward was so intense I couldn't walk, or even move, really.

I'll never, ever forget how it felt like every cell in my body was vigorously vibrating with a heightened sense of ecstasy.

We'll start with the Desire song of sex, because this song is widely misunderstood, misused, and has been slaughtered by the righteous minds of many religions and governing bodies.

There MUST be a desire for sex.

We may either try to eradicate it or over-indulge in it, but whatever the case, this song only cares about one thing: *the full, innocent, untethered expression of your sexual being.*

Please note this does not solely refer to the act of sex, our sexuality is profound. It has the potential to ignite one of the greatest mysteries we know: the creation of life. A mystery that belongs to nature, one that she abundantly expresses—and yet, even nature's fecundity doesn't diminish the awe we feel in the presence of new life: like the gardener with her plants, a musician with his music, the intensity of springtime and the overflowing grace of autumn, not to mention the endless births that occur in each new moment: new creations are awesome.

To be clear, our sexuality isn't a commodity—something for us to trade and bargain with. Our sexuality is our own aliveness—*it's the animating force within us as well as all living beings.*

The desire for sex is a song as old as existence. This song lives beneath the calculating eye of all of our scientific and mathematical formulas and theories about life. Without Eros, there would be no life.

"When Eros leaves, he takes the heart with him. Eros is not just a principle of relatedness, but the very embodiment of desire and sensuality. Without the erotic sensibility that he confers, the delight in the sensual world, the love he inspires, and the desire he instills -- for he is, himself, a potent mix of all these -- the heart fails."

Lyn Cowan

Desire for sex is essential, but the problem lies in sex becoming a currency, one that even the poorest person can use to cash in. This is far off the mark.

We do not understand the potency of our own aliveness; we can't seem to grasp it beyond "trade" or "procreation." We've forgotten the original meaning of this sacred song: *when desire for sex sings within your body it is NOT A SIGNAL TO HAVE SEX, it's a signal of activation, of being switched-on and that is enough!*

I walked in front of him, down a hill we'd just hiked. He'd kissed me at the top and I could still feel his lips on mine.

Behind me, his presence filled the space, so much so that purple and blue spots swirled in my vision as I quickened my pace.

It would have been so easy to have sex up there, but we didn't. We just breathed each other in.

Now, as we were heading back to the car, I was having a perpetual orgasm. Every step I took felt like I was stroking the depths of my desire, and waves upon waves of deep pleasure cascaded through me.

Giddy, I surrendered, allowing my turn-on to take over, letting my heart race in the fullness of my yearning. In that moment, I was making love to everything around me.

Primarily this song connects us with our right relationship, to the fecundity of life. In this state, we become more healthy, creative, and magnetic. In fact, there are many accounts of ancient cultures understanding this premise and building entire systems of practice and meditation to pay homage to this potent capacity within each of us.

How do we bridge the gap between either our irreverence about or our addiction to this song, and its actual offering?

Shame and Desire

Let's first start with the role of shame.

Since each of us is born shameless, we must actually learn shame, which is an integral part of the virus—the illness of domestication.

Shame is designed to make us behave in particular ways. Shame around the desire for sex is designed to stop us from partaking in any form of it —and if we do still partake, it ensures we feel bad about our experience afterward.

Shame is useless, it implies we do not trust ourselves to make choices, to have natural morality, to know our self-respect and respect for others.

Because of shame, we are conditioned to mistrust the song of desire for sex and, therefore, we move further and further away from feeling healthy, creative, and magnetic.

If you trade your authenticity for safety, you may experience the following: anxiety, depression, eating disorders, addiction, rage, blame, resentment, and inexplicable grief. ~ Brené Brown, Shame Researcher

Shame is at the heart of illness, especially that of our mind. Shame births neurosis and sexually neurotic people are unhealthy, uncreative hungry ghosts. They can hurt themselves and/or others in their attempt to resolve their neurosis. Within each of us, we have a knowing of how to be in right relationship with our own sexuality.

Unfortunately, we inherit the shame of our lineage, which is then further indoctrinated through consensual reality—the group agreement about how things are. For example, priests who preach purity and celibacy and then turn around and sexually abuse children.

We wrongly blame desire, we make her into a demon of ill intent, but desire is pure. She is the voice of our soul, calling us deeper into aliveness. It's shame that destroys and confuses the original song, skewing its meaning so only neurosis can be expressed. Therefore, it's shame we must address in order to start our journey back into our own state of erotic innocence.

I've come to understand that Eros is evolutionary and that each one of us is right where we naturally need to be. Understanding where we are in our erotic evolution is central to liberating ourselves and accessing the fullness of our ever-emerging, ever-evolving Desire.

STAGE ONE: EROTIC INNOCENCE

We are all born pure, free, and shameless.

We know without knowing that we belong to life and the sensation of aliveness feels exquisite and is completely natural, similar to breathing. We know without knowing that our own sexuality is simply part of the whole—not segregated and reserved for fickle acts, but an integral part of expressing ourselves.

We enjoy our bodies because they are designed, by nature, to be enjoyable. Touch is a sensation that elicits aliveness, as do all of our senses. In fact, our sensuality is how we learn to *make sense of reality*.

As an innocent, there is no part of our body we cannot touch and enjoy, including the assigned sexual parts. In truth, the pleasure we later reserve for our genitals is originally experienced throughout our entire body.

Innocence (or "in-no-sense") has no need to judge the world by polarizing it into good/

bad, right/wrong, etc. Rather, it takes in every experience as a whole, digesting it completely and translating it through the sexual, felt-sense of our being.

When we are in innocence, we are wide open, porous, and profoundly receptive. In fact, in the first five years of our lives our brain is in a perpetual hypnotic state, allowing for a fuller intake of the world. This is an organic design to ensure we absorb as much as we can for our survival.

It's through this hypnosis that we, undiscerning, absorb everything around us: the first (necessary) elements of domestication sets in. In this phase of our evolution, our innocence enables us to learn far faster than at any other phase in our lifespan, but we have not yet developed a capacity for wisdom—which emerges organically from partaking in our life's experiences.

When it comes to the song of sexuality, erotic innocence serves to call us back into right relationship with the truth about our sexuality.

We are born omni-orgasmic beings. Orgasms are the experience of our inborn aliveness in its actual form. It isn't random: it's how life feels when it's fully present.

For most of us, however, an orgasm is either nonexistent or is only a fleeting, temporary source of pleasure, ending more in frustration than in satisfaction. For a tiny second, we feel whole, free, healthy, connected—and then it's over.

Yet, when we were omni-orgasmic, we were in a perpetual unfolding of aliveness, vitality and freedom. All things external and all parts of us could elicit this connection.

We are, in actuality, unlimited in our resource of life. However, very quickly, the virus of domestication—socialized conditioning—is spread and we lose this enlivening orientation to life and ourselves.

We learn that touching ourselves is bad—and attracting the touch of others is bad, scary, and possibly very harmful—so we doubt and we lay the discordant tone of shame upon our unblemished song of sexual desire.

In this stage, we are wide open to and highly influenced by the opinions and habits of our parents or main caregivers.

My mother shared with me, pretty much from birth, how to self-pleasure. Not as in showing me techniques and the how-tos, but through being relaxed and spacious about my own curiosity and self-exploration. In other words, she never shamed me.

Luckily for me, both she and my father had chosen, before my birth, to create a safe and loving container for natural sexuality to exist for their children, as they did not wish to pass on the strict Catholic views that were beaten into both of them as they grew up in French Canada.

Therefore, I would delight in my own body pretty much anywhere and at anytime, as though it was the most natural and obvious thing for me to do.

Rather than shaming me, my parents set clear boundaries of where it was appropriate for me to enjoy myself, while also making it clear that no adult should ever touch me, period.

STAGE TWO: EROTIC ACTIVATION

Just to make things even more highly concentrated, our small, young bodies are suddenly flooded with a new intensity—massive levels of hormones! This huge influx changes us physically, emotionally, and mentally. It's been said that teens suffer from "hormonally induced insanity" due to the exceptionally high levels of hormones coursing through their developing bodies.

In this stage of our erotic evolution, we suddenly grasp that sexuality is a powerful force. We don't yet fully grasp why, we only know it's an intense subject that everyone has an opinion about.

Moreover, our social conditioning makes it clear that our sexuality is a viable currency, something we can use to get something. For example, young teen women trading blow jobs for homework assignments.

This further skews our song of sexual desire, adding layers of shame, abuse, conditioning, and assumptions. There are few who escape this.

Yet, in the few that do, a beautiful, relaxed, natural relationship develops with one's own body and pleasure. Our psyche is relaxed, while our Eros is freely and innocently explored. For the most part, these rare free individuals do not partake in sexual games, but rather they are relaxed, and self-contained, not needing anything from others.

After my severe burn accident, I did not feel attractive and withdrew into a very insular, hermit-like lifestyle.

At the time I was also in my first year of home schooling and dedicated to time-intensive dance training, so this absorbed most of my social time.

My sexual relationship with myself did not stop. In fact, a month after my first period, I began to ejaculate during my orgasms. It was a fantastic new addition to my expanding pleasure.

I was also observing the drama and dissatisfaction of my girlfriends with their teen boyfriends and concluded early on that I would not bother being sexual with anyone until I was old enough to be sexual with an adult man.

I decided to avoid heartache and also gain the benefit of knowing my own body and pleasure through remaining single. This also meant that by the time I was of legal age, and took my first lover, I had mind-blowing, pain-free, multi-orgasmic sex from that first time onward.

We rarely teach our teens about pleasure: rather, we infect their minds with all the problems, diseases, and evil that can come with sexuality, which further compounds their growing mistrust and misunderstanding of the very natural song of sexual desire.

However, it was not always this way. In cultures of old, it was understood that young people needed to learn about their sexuality and how to make love in satisfying ways. Take the old traditions in Uganda, where young women were taught by their aunt, the art of self-pleasure—for the purpose of enhancing pleasure with another.

"Experts locally known as Ssenga, a title meaning 'paternal aunt,' and broadly used to refer to women specializing in sex education, say that three fingers are used to pull each of the lips downwards for several weeks."

"Psychological benefits have also sustained the practice. To women, it builds confidence and self-esteem to look like other women in Buganda."

"These and many other benefits have made Okukyalira ensiko, which literally means visiting the bush, an integral part of sex baptism among Uganda's largest ethnic group."

"Far from promoting promiscuity. as one ignorant European writer claims, the tradition prepares girls for what society considers the most enjoyable and most pleasurable form of lovemaking."

"In fact, one of Kampala's leading Ssenga, told me that European women have started coming to her to have their labia minora elongated. The people of the West would certainly learn a lot from Africa if they overcame their bigotry..."

"[E]ncoded within the Ssenga institution, [is] enhanced sexual pleasure for women, and expanded...perceptions of themselves as active sexual beings."

"Imagine a world where our sensual nature was not demonized, but cultivated and refined."

Yahya Sseremba

Unfortunately, we are so afraid of this song of desire and sex that we contaminate the lives of our young adults in this stage of erotic evolution.

In the state of erotic activation, we are still very much under the influence of our peers, whatever media we have access to, and the opinions of authority figures in our life.

STAGE THREE: EROTIC EXPLORATION

In this phase of our erotic evolution, it's natural to be curious and to explore all of our available sexual options. We tend to seek out learning through readily available media, books, and, of course, porn.

We learn what we like and don't like, and develop a degree of confidence and skill in the bedroom.

If an individual ignores this exploratory phase or is forbidden from it, their erotic evolution stagnates, and they can develop a neurotic relationship with desire and sex.

If we can relax, be curious, and just allow ourselves the freedom to experiment, we'll soon discover what is true for us without having to make it good/bad, right/wrong, kinky/vanilla, etc.

Our Eros doesn't care for boxes and definitions; she only cares if we express ourselves.

Often, however, we can get caught up in this stage, through an addiction or an aversion to it. In an addiction scenario, we may believe porn, and/or other external sources of sexual education/exploration, is the end-all and be-all of our sexuality. We may imagine that without such influences, sex would be boring.

Addiction can lead to a loss of pleasure and satisfaction, such as in the case of young men addicted to porn and Viagra. Their self-pleasure gets more and more extreme as their experience of pleasure becomes more and more fleeting. Loaded with expectations and performance anxiety, they become increasingly reluctant to seek out an actual sexual experience with a real person. Therefore, the cycle continues, until the day they choose to stop it.

Aversion works in opposition to addiction, but is equally painful and dissatisfying. With aversion, we are afraid to touch the edges of our desire and to allow ourselves, even if purely in the realm of fantasy, the spaciousness to explore something unusual or novel.

This can form imposed aversion as well, such as saving oneself for marriage. In this case, vagina-penis sex is avoided at all costs, but anal and oral sex is used to release the sexual tension that arises in healthy humans. Whatever the case, aversion is often loaded and led by shame.

True sexual exploration occurs outside of this polarity. It's as natural as breathing—and for some, this stage of erotic evolution brings a sense of what is true for themselves and a relaxation into whatever orientation most completes their unique individuality.

Needless to say, in this stage, we are still externally focused on our learning and orientation, even though we are free to sift through and absorb a massive amount of sexual "how to" information.

My first real boyfriend was a man who had been with the same woman from the age of fourteen to twenty-three. He had known no other woman.

I met him at a party where I was making my rounds, enjoying the deliciousness of multiple sensual experiences, exploring the unique nuances of how each new person kissed.

When my lips met his, the world stopped for a moment and all else disappeared.

This was the beginning of an intense sexual connection, one where we'd have, on average, eight hours of sex every day! Because he was so fresh to the world of epic sex, he was intensely curious, and I was very experienced already at twenty-one years of age, I agreed to an adventurous, erotic exploration.

Probably our sweetest exploration was before we'd ever actually made love. We connected with a mutual gay friend who was very into my boyfriend and had admitted he would enjoy exploring me as well.

A very innocent three-way exploration emerged, one involving no intercourse, but everything else. I was amazed and fascinated at all the possibilities and discovered that when it comes to Eros, traditional male-female roles made no sense.

STAGE FOUR: EROTIC EXPANSION

This is an intriguing stage, because it's the point where mechanistic sex is no longer fulfilling or fascinating. It's the point where we start to feel, *there must be more to sex than this.* And we are right—there is!

During this stage of our erotic evolution, we may become aware of and genuinely pursue, the more spiritual versions of sexuality, such as Tantra, the Taoist sexual arts, and any form of conscious sexuality. These practices, in general, encourage more connection with our partners and ourselves, a slowing down of the act of sex, a refinement of how to give and receive pleasure, and a prolonging of the sexual experience.

These traditions encourage both solo and partnered cultivation practices, which hopefully are inclusive of our hearts. I say "hopefully," because although most of these traditional "spiritual-sexual" approaches have tremendous value for an evolving sexuality, they are still limited by the capacity and integrity of their teacher. It's unfortunately all too common that they impose just as much dogma as society imposes on the "less-spiritual" version of sexuality.

Thankfully, this phase does invite us to continue in expanding our own definitions of pleasure and sex to include spirituality. Yet, as in the previous three stages, in this fourth stage, we are still subject to external referencing, under the continued influence of spiritual sexuality gurus, who define our sexuality by their own indoctrinated viewpoint.

I wasn't at all in the mood to make love, but my husband slowly kissed my feet and moved up my body, always conscious of simply letting me feel adored.

After a long time under his devotional attention, I felt myself open up, like a flower opens to drink in the heat of the sun.

What came from our union shocked me. There we were, in a basic hotel room, yet I was literally seeing the cosmos swirling in his skin!

Every time I touched him, galaxies spun, nebulas undulated, and tears of immense awe flowed from my eyes.

God was making love with me.

STAGE FIVE: EROTIC WISDOM

This is the final stage of our erotic evolution and it's where we come full circle. We return to erotic innocence, only this time we have the experience and wisdom of an adult mind and heart. We return to the truth—that we are sexual "beings," not just sexual "doings."

We are both now innocent and wise in our orientation with desire and our expression of sexuality. We understand that shame is useless and we discard it.

We get that being turned on means being alive. We get that we are truly omni-orgasmic and we experience life this way again.

We enjoy being relaxed in our desire and we are free to enjoy sexual tension for the sake of its scintillating delight. We no longer feel an urgency to collude with consensual reality: rather, we exercise our sexual sovereignty. We are at ease, in a state of erotic grace.

Unfortunately, there are few living examples of this particular state of our erotic evolution. Most of what is available to us is the second & third stages, with a sprinkle of the fourth. Yet, all of the preceding stages are still important, as evolutionary stages require external feedback and orientation.

In this fifth stage, in which we are self-sourced and self-defined, we finally come home to ourselves as true sexual beings and finally, unfetter ourselves from the habits and opinions of others and return to our own inner knowing, as our compass.

This stage can be terrifying for many, since it requires 100 percent responsibility and accountability. We no longer can make external things or people responsible for our sexual experiences, whether they let us down or bring us to our leading edge of pleasure.

This stage is essential to our own evolution. Regardless of the lack of living examples, we can still emerge in our sexual sovereignty and abide in the totality of our enlivenment.

I'd been celibate for more than a year, yet fully devoted to my solo-cultivation. On this particular night, I lay back after my breast massage and ovarian breathing, to absorb the champagne-like bubbles that were moving through me.

It was in the quietude of my meditation that it began: a deep, slow wave of the most ecstatic proportions.

Orgasms layered themselves one after another, the last more epic than the preceding. In fact, I became hyperconscious and so incredibly expanded that at some point I recognized I was having what could only be labeled as, a cosmic orgasm—the immensity of it beyond anything I'd yet experienced.

It left me wholly fulfilled and complete and wondering how I'd ever go back to having sex with another person.

BEING WHERE WE ARE

All of us are where we are; there is no stage of erotic evolution that is better to be in than another. Each stage carries important aspects of our erotic genius.

We must remember the purity of our desire; the glorious beauty of this song, without the cacophony shame can bring to it.

We get to love where we are, allowing ourselves to relax into it and know that no matter where we are on our sexual journey, it's an important and essential part of our life.

If we are dissatisfied with how it's been or currently is, this is a perfect moment to pause, notice and to ask ourselves: Am I in a relationship with the pure song of my desire for sex or am I relating to my sexuality from a contrived, conditioned, and collusive orientation?

If we've never considered trusting our own desire, then we have come to a beautiful cross-road on our journey: choosing to lean into our natural erotic edges or not: and to be curious about our own desire song or not.

The choice has always been and will always be ours to make.

Chapter 4

The Desire Song of Love

The hunger for love is much more difficult to remove than the hunger for bread.

Mother Theresa

After the annulment of my first marriage, I never thought I'd love again. My heart had been ripped into a million pieces and I feared it would never quite be functional again.

Yet, time did its work on me, and a few years later I found myself listening to the beating of my heart and I heard her whisper:

"I'm ready. I'm ready to know unconditional love."

And so, again, I allowed myself to open up and very soon afterward, I met the man who would become my second husband, and who, despite my objections, would provide me with the most excruciating lessons in being unconditional with my love.

Love Enlivens All Things

The Desire for love is an achingly beautiful desire, it's a part of being a human being, a unique mammalian orientation to life.

Consider the desire song for love as the glue, the teacher, the guide, the salve, and the fuel for the nourishment of our essence.

Without love—in its truest sense—the world feels alien, harsh, cold, scary, cruel, and hopeless. Think of love as the warm current that enlivens all things great and beautiful within the human spirit. Consider our understanding of love as a state of being through the lens of ancient Grecian culture. Love was so important to the Greeks of old that they created six unique words to describe love: *eros, "sexual passion," philia, "deep friendship," ludus, "playful love," agape, "love of everyone," pragma "longstanding love," & philautia, "love of the self."*

The celebration of love in its exalted form was made obvious through the worship of Aphrodite, the goddess of love and beauty, and the presence of the great Aphrodite temples, which refined the arts of love and beauty.

In fact, it's interesting to note that it was in this culture that marriage rites originated. Couples would seek the blessing of Aphrodite, to make a sacred offering of their love to the goddess herself.

Socialized Love

However, the true desire song of love is no longer culturally understood, let alone exalted. For the most part, as much as we all feel the deep yearning for love, we associate love with great pain. This form of love is the hijacked version of this desire song.

Love was never intended to be a socially mandated, conditional demand that we make of another. This version of love is what lies hidden behind jealousy, revenge, hate, rage, cruelty, and all things ugly in our human behavior. This impoverished version of love is what we're all indoctrinated into from very early on in life.

It would be honest to say that this form of socialized love is demonic as it distorts our original and true desire to express and receive love into something that is quite shallow, empty and manipulative.

The key essential component of love—profound respect for self, others and Life—is what is missing from this hijacked version of the desire song for love.

"When conditional love dominates the Dream of the Planet, any semblance of peace and harmony occurs through force, when one person or persons, subjugate the will of others."

Don Miguel Ruiz Jr.

Hijacked love is everywhere.

Think of all the ways we are currently conditional with ourselves and with others in our life. And all the ways they are with us, conditional love is really all most of us know. Unconditional love—the true desire song of love—is perhaps felt as a possibility, but not as a knowing.

To know something, to have true gnosis, we must have a direct experience of it. It's fair to say that few of us have had a direct experience of love that comes without any conditions.

Some will argue a mother's love is unconditional, but that's not exactly true. Along with her love comes a million and one conditions that she has for her child, and when those are not met, she may withdraw her love.

This initial withdrawing of love feels utterly terrifying to a young child, like a death threat. This is how we quickly learn what our mother wants from us. How we should behave to get rewarded with her love, and the pain of consistently disappointing her and falling short of her ideals for us.

This isn't the fault of our mother, she is just as domesticated as we are: she is simply putting into practice all the conditions she learned from her childhood and beyond. Yes, she may have good intentions to change a few of those conditions, but inevitably, there are conditions to her love.

Therefore, we learn this is what love is, and our natural desire song of love is hijacked. This is such a deep imprint, that we may fail to recognize any other versions of love that come our way.

"Who we are and who we become depends, in part, on whom we love."

Thomas Lewis

This desire song for love is so crucial to both our survival and thriving in life. It's essential that we keep our heart wide open, no matter how battered we may feel by the experience of hijacked love.

My husband lost his mother to cancer, and in the process, I lost my husband to his depression.

That's why when I met Tim; I was shocked to experience something utterly unexpected. We sat in front of each other, in a meditation group, and as our eyes met, my world expanded into the incomprehensible vastness of what Tim calls, "big love".

I felt seen and I was seeing. I felt as though there were no boundaries, no stories, no limitations, and no restrictions—in fact, all there was in that moment was the immensity of a vast and deep ocean of love.

The starved and shriveled parts of me lit up, renewed and refueled in ways I never knew possible—with someone I hardly knew.

To this day, when I connect with Tim, even over Skype, I immediately enter the flow-state of "big love," and suddenly the entire world feels brighter, fuller, and more magical.

What's gorgeous in this desire song for love is that it's intrinsically part of who we are, which is why we feel so drawn to expressing the fullness of our natural love and to receive the same from another expressed human heart.

And what's equally gorgeous is this desire for love remains available to us no matter how entangled we are in the hijacked version of love. The second we turn our attention to our own living truth—that love is who we are naturally—we immediately feel the experience of its potent warmth.

In fact, it's so potent, so disarming, so vulnerable, few of us can stand being in the presence of this love. We may quickly attempt to diminish this desire song and replace it with something much more familiar and far more conditional.

"Each of us has an inner thermostat setting that determines how much love, success, and creativity we allow ourselves to enjoy. When we exceed our inner thermostat setting, we will often do something to sabotage ourselves, causing us to drop back into the old, familiar zone where we feel secure."

Gay Hendricks, PhD

The Beggar and the Gourmet

When I'm facilitating a workshop with women, one of the most commonly asked questions is about love—specifically, now that they are learning new levels of self-love, how this will translate into loving others.

This is where I bring in the idea of the beggar and gourmet orientations to relationships. In the beggar orientation, one who has learned and adopted the ideals of hijacked love, we naturally bargain for love, including exchanging sex for the hopes of keeping love. We wrongly believe someone else needs to fill our beggar's bowl.

This kind of love is impoverished from the start as it assumes we are not complete to begin with, that we require the presence of another to complete ourselves, and furthermore, that we are not worthy of receiving love as we are and must learn to compromise ourselves so everyone can be happy.

This is a very common and socially acceptable form of love. In fact, people often refer to their partner as their "better half."

In a gourmet orientation to relationships, we are whole unto ourselves. We have returned to a state of deep self-love and self-fulfillment, and we recognize that relationships are purely for celebration and for creating a life together.

Here we have intact "non-negotiables" (the values in our lives that hold meaning and integrity, that we are not willing to bargain away). We come into a relationship full and ready to share abundantly and generously, curious about the equally generous offering that another gourmet individual is open to sharing with us.

Here we are in the natural expression of the true desire song of love, one where we deeply respect each other. In fact, having profound respect for others and ourselves is a clear indication of being in the true desire song of love.

When respect is missing, we are guaranteed to be living out the hijacked version of love.

Coming Home to Our Own Hearts

The key to being able to enjoy and cultivate the true desire song of love and experience the profundity of what unconditional love has to offer is to first come home to our own hearts.

We are all heartsick. Every single person of the modern, domesticated world, suffers from a heart condition, in which the true nature of our hearts is distorted through the sickness of hijacked love.

In the rare remaining tribes that are isolated in the deep wilderness of the world, we can still witness the true desire song of love singing, unrestricted in everyone, young and old alike.

I was sitting on a freshly cut log when the children arrived. The eldest came straight over to me and plunked a five month old into my lap. The baby's deep brown eyes looked into mine—relaxed, open, and trusting—and we remained in this intimate connection for well over half an hour.

Not once did the baby struggle, fidget or complain, but rather she seemed very curious about who I was, allowing her tiny, warm body to melt into the softness of my breasts and belly.

The rest of my group was in awe, simply observing this rare phenomenon, knowing that back home, babies would never be carried by children, let alone put into the lap of a complete stranger.

However, deep in the Amazon, these tribal kids did more to heal our hearts than all our other efforts combined.

Spending even as little as a few days with these undomesticated people, has a profound impact on our own hearts, as we quickly begin to remember what it's like to be true to our own nature.

Our initial offer of hijacked love doesn't fool any of them. They don't bargain for love, but rather, openly offer up their unbridled openness.

Upon returning from such "primitive" cultures, we are hit with the prevalence of heart-sickness within every single person we meet. It is excruciating to return to this world of hijacked love with the felt understanding of our real potential for love.

The good news is love can and does exist in healthy ways, and each one of us has the power to cultivate this form of love in our day-to-day lives.

As with the other desire songs, the return to the true calling of our hearts is always just one choice away.

Chapter 5

The Desire Song of Procreation

"The longer you wait for something, the more you'll appreciate it when you get it. Because anything worth having is definitely worth waiting for."

Anonymous

They lost their first baby and couldn't get pregnant again. Time was running out as they were both in their forties and desperate to start a family.

That's how they found themselves in the heart of the Sequoia tribe, searching for healing that could possibly bring into the world, the expression of their deepest union.

Being a part of those ceremonies, I was witness to both their resistance to surrendering to the Shaman's invitations and to the direct experience of sensing the profound presence of their daughter—a light so brilliant I could not turn my eyes toward her.

A year later, when they called to invite me to their blessing way (a ceremony to celebrate the arrival of their daughter), I felt I had to be there—since, in some way, I felt I had been part of their conscious conception.

Resting my hands on the fullness of her belly and seeing the love radiating from her eyes, I knew the desire for pregnancy and the beauty of bringing forth a child who is truly desired and truly loved.

I used to think that the desire to have children was more of a woman's thing, but it's not true. Men equally desire to sire their own progeny.

We attribute this particular desire song to nature and encourage it, for the most part. However, sometimes we take this encouragement a little too far—and then it becomes an expectation, another facet of domestication, and another collusive agreement. This is how the pressure builds; the shaming builds, the guilt builds, and unconscious coupling ensues.

Unconsciously creating humans is not the solution to an overpopulated planet, so how does this particular desire song, the desire for family, come to serve the greater good?

Our Creation Song

This song is ancient, older than the beginning, since it must be sung for any beginning to occur. This song is our creation song, not only did our parents hear it, we also heard and responded to its call.

It's a pure song, a song of mystery, a song that opens a portal, allowing life to emerge where none existed. Its potency is beyond measure, imagine this pure creative force that can literally create something from nothing, that can spark another being into physicality? It's a miracle!

This song is the song of living miracles and we are all touched by it, or we wouldn't exist. For eons, this song has birthed stars, planets, insects, trees, and more recently, humans. However, what happens when the song is played with a filter? When obligation and the compulsion to comply with social constructs kick starts us on a journey of creating a family? What happens when it's not consciously chosen?

This song cares for only one thing: the creation of life.

It doesn't care about the conditions or neurosis of those touched by it. It's a song that never stops singing, so what's really going on?

In consciousness, when this song is sung, we surrender to it and experience conscious choice in the process of life creation. Many people have shared that they "knew" when they conceived, that they "felt" it.

Yet, now our choice to sing along with creation remains, for the most part, unconscious, hijacked by our domestication. Some of us actually believe we will be "more of a woman" once we have children, or that getting married means we must start a family.

Or, in some circumstances, we unconsciously let our conditioning blind us in our pursuit of love, when what's actually motivating us is an urge, an impulse, a genuine desire to create life—in other words, our desire to create a family can convince us to pursue love.

"We are survival machines – robot vehicles blindly programmed to preserve the selfish molecules known as genes. This is a truth which still fills me with astonishment."

Richard Dawkins

This song is tricky when tampered with.

It's easy to hijack this natural urge.

Too many children are born to parents who resent them, who are absent, who do not have the time, means, emotional maturity, and presence to properly respect this fresh new life. And so we perpetuate our wounding and misery.

In some cultures, disrespect begins with the first breath an infant takes, especially if it's a girl. An unspoken agreement ripples through the room: *It's too bad she's not a boy...*

We do not respect the gift of this song: we allow ourselves to be swayed by outer pressures and lose touch with how precious life is.

For some of us, who are honest, we never really feel the urge to bind and flow with this particular song of desire for family. For us, this song is gently in the background, inspiring us to birth other things, in other ways, as a way to contribute to the act of creation.

This desire song is potent, ceaseless, and eternal. Choosing to consciously sing this song requires us to first shed all of our conditions and to return to a state in which this choice is truly a conscious one, and not the result of social and religious pressures.

Having reverence for this unique life mystery enables us to choose the path of conscious conception, the only place where both, pro-life and pro-choice views get to meet in respectful agreement.

Chapter 6

The Desire Song of Rapture

"The universe began, not with light, but with Desire, 'the primal seed and germ of Spirit'."

Hindu Rig Veda (second millennium BC)

The hypocrisy of religion didn't escape my eight-year-old mind. I experienced this realization when my parents finally succumbed to my insistent demand we go to church on Sunday. They had avoided church, because for them, it was a painful reminder of their indoctrination.

Not only did I have to sit through boring, meaningless words, while wild birds flew freely in the sky outside the church windows, I was also not allowed to go up for the special treat and juice that everyone else was allowed to enjoy.

On top of that, our neighbor, who was sexually abusing all of his children and beating his wife on a daily basis, was sitting in front of us, praying to his God.

My young heart could not make sense of such discrepancies, so —to my parents' relief—I said I'd never go back to church again.

Yet, every single night, I would look skyward and pray to my beloved that was somewhere out in the great cosmos, and every night, I'd fall asleep with reverence, filling my heart with devotional love.

This desire song is connected to our spiritual pursuits and religious inclinations and can best be understood through the quality of rapture.

Rapture derives from its obsolete French meaning: "seizing and carrying off," a sense that the religious of old felt, they were "transported" to their God. While a mere sporadic verse on the lips of disciples, rapture is a common song amongst the great saints and enlightened ones. Rapture occurs when our desire to know God is expressed.

This is when true *gnosis* (knowledge through direct experience) appears, when we come home to our maker and understand our place in the scheme of life and the universe.

To say there is a desire song in spirituality (and even in religion) may be blasphemy to some, but what calls us to God/Goddess/Buddha/Allah/Creator? What pulls us to deeply yearn to know this?

Desire.

The Fragrance of Rapture

"I once had a thousand desires. But in my one Desire to know you all else melted away."

Rumi

This song of rapture is the ecstasy of divine union we hear of and yearn for. Some of us believe that this is the only righteous song.

Many of us do not freely choose our religious/spiritual orientation. It's indoctrinated into us through parental, familial, and tribal systems. To choose an orientation in opposition with it can mean certainty of death in some circumstances. Some of us do not follow our own calling, our own pure song of spiritual desire. Instead, we emptily follow the herd, going through rote rituals in hopes to have the promised rapture—but rarely, if ever, do we taste its sweet nectar.

However, when this song is remembered in its purity and followed with pure devotion, rapture is not only felt, it becomes the state of being that we constantly live in.

Remember the omni-orgasmic state? Its fragrance is very close to rapture. This is why, in their true, unconditioned forms, the desire for sex & the desire for rapture are not polar opposites, but counterparts in the greater symphony of our life.

For me, the wilderness is my spirituality. It's the place I feel closest to life, it's the place where I shed my domestication and remember rapture. Simply sitting upon a rock's ledge, in awakened stillness, I experience rapture. Suddenly, I'm part of all living beings, a part of the fabric of life.

Occasionally in life there are those moments of unutterable fulfillment, which cannot be completely explained by those symbols called words. Their meanings can only be articulated by the inaudible language of the heart.

Martin Luther King, Jr.

Whatever our Spiritual orientation, we do it disservice if we bind this desire song with righteous rhetoric.

Rapture can only be heard by those who choose their path with every fiber of their being, who devote their moments to the greater mystery and who open themselves to the humbling and ecstatic beauty of what is too profound for words to touch.

I've been touched by rapture in the most unexpected moments. One specific time was when the sunset, in all its glorious splendor, did more than just illuminate the sky, it touched my very core.

As I let myself surrender to the beauty, a wave of omni-orgasmic delight exploded inside me and I found myself flowing with ambrosia as I orgasmed over and over again, purely by the sight of this natural phenomena.

Chapter 7

The Desire Song of Thriving

And in the end it's not the years in your life
that count. It's the life in your years.

Abraham Lincoln

"Make me stop..." Her voice so quiet, I wasn't sure I'd heard her correctly.

It was 3:37a.m. the night darker than black, and this sudden shock of reality rattled me awake. "I'm here," I croaked, trying to soften my anxiety into reassurance.

She'd never called me like this before. Many times I had assisted my friend through deep bouts of intense depression, but this time I could feel, even over the phone, the razor's edge pressing into the pulsing vein of her lifeline.

I forced away the fuzziness of sleep—no amount of joking or sweet talk was going to work this time. No, this time, I could sense a terrifying and imminent threat hanging over us, like the silent pause before the downswing of a samurai's sword.

"I was just about to do it...then you came into my thoughts... so I called." Her words stumbled out like fractals on a bad LSD trip.

"I'm glad you called. I'm here and I'm not going anywhere. Let me be with you." I found my center, despite my racing heart. She's attempting to kill herself! This isn't a nightmare it's real! My head was reeling as the harshness of the truth hit my waking mind.

"I've tried, but what's the point? I'll never be good enough, sexy enough, desirable enough, or acceptable enough. I'm tired; I'm tired of trying. It never leads to anything anyways. I hate my life and I hate myself. I can't even breathe right now I'm so depressed." She was attempting to convince me to let her take her own life.

This was the start of a long, arduous call, one that, at any instant, could have turned from scary to profoundly tragic.

Survival First

Survival is primal—it's the urgency to wake up and take action now or roll over and die. This creates strong adrenaline in acute cases and an overdose of cortisol in chronic cases.

Every living being does its best to find equilibrium. If our lives are extremely unbalanced, we'll never hear the song of desire to thrive. We'll be preoccupied with the alarm bell eroding our sensitive system—and if we cannot find equilibrium fairly quickly, then we may actually give up on fully living our life.

It's interesting to note that even when individuals suffer from inhumane conditions—a life of trauma and PTSD (in war zones, for example)—there can be moments when our true nature shines, when the desire to thrive lets us know we can.

"When women first come they cannot see you, they can't talk to you, they are ashamed, they are fearful, but after six months at City of Joy they can stand, talk without fear, without shame, and they have confidence in themselves."

Francine Bintu

What does thriving mean to us when so many of us, even those far more blessed and fortunate, are stuck in the perpetual cycle of survival?

To Thrive, Not Just Survive

To thrive is to make the most out of our moments. When our attention is on grace: gratitude for being alive, for having a healthy body, for having a place to sleep, for the gift of a simple meal, and so forth.

It's also the joy of expression: when we are freed from our tunnel vision and find wonderment in the vast nuances of every moment. We take in four hundred billion bits of information *per second* and yet we are only ever consciously aware of about two thousand of those bits. This tiny bandwidth doesn't leave room for the profundity of life.

In February of 1994, I found myself waking up from an emergency laparoscopy surgery, where small incisions are made in order to look inside you with a camera.

"You have two weeks to live. Better contact your family and set your affairs straight," my surgeon told me dispassionately.

I blinked, not quite sure I'd heard her right, did she just say I was going to die in two weeks?! An overwhelming mix of disbelief and panic churned in my belly.

I immediately called my mother and a shaman friend I knew as "Uncle" and relayed the tragic news. They both surprised me by laughing and recommending I do the same.

So in the face of death, I laughed and I chose to live.

I proceeded to defy my doctor's diagnosis and started down a long road, from surviving a violent rape, to emerging an inspired, thriving woman.

I remain grateful for this powerful moment in my life because it's when my journey on the path of conscious sexuality began—and the rest is history.

Even in the worst life-threatening moments, there can be a choice, against all odds: the choice to thrive (not just survive). This is the song that not only leads us out of survival—it invites us into the creative experience of thriving.

Anyone of us can choose.

I've seen the poorest of people—although they had nothing—relish their moments, their eyes afire with a beautiful sparkle, their laughter coming easily, their playfulness unmistakable. In fact, in my opinion, they had real wealth: good friends, fresh air, simple, open moments unburdened by the complexity of our modern times.

Thriving is simple.

It's not *stuff* it's an *attitude.*

It's the desire to make the most out of every moment, while experiencing gratitude and wonderment. We are all just one choice away from having just that.

I once met an older gentleman at an airport, he was so full of life that I was drawn to ask him what his secret was.

He replied with a grin, "I don't sweat the small stuff."

"Ah," I replied. I was wondering what qualified for him as "small stuff" when he leaned forward and whispered playfully, "And it's ALL small stuff!"

I was reeling at the possibility, could it all really be just that simple?

I've contemplated these words for a long time and have come to see that this is, indeed, the secret to thriving! It's liberating to know it really is "all small stuff."

This doesn't negate or belittle any of our challenges, but rather, it places them in the context of the greater scheme of things. Even those facing death get to choose whether to shut down and miss out on the beauty of their remaining days, or make the most of every precious second they have left.

This desire song can become like our favorite soundtrack from an inspirational movie. It's very memorable: once we hear it we may find ourselves humming it unconsciously. The choice to sing this song is ever-present, a choice we get to play with every day of our short lives.

Chapter 8

The Desire Song of Contribution

There are certain things that are fundamental to human fulfillment. The essence of these needs is captured in the phrase 'to live, to love, to learn, to leave a legacy.' The need to leave a legacy is our spiritual need to have a sense of meaning, purpose, personal congruence, and contribution.

Steven R. Covey

My grandfather came from a large, and extremely poor family of twelve kids. Although he had nothing, he always had the spirit of contribution.

In a time when few people were free, he'd been a true entrepreneur. Owning more than a hundred female horses to cultivate Premarin for a local doctor's birth control project, to running a delivery business, and starting up a local grocery store that provided for an entire village.

When he retired, his need to contribute continued. He built a small hobby farm and supplied our family with raw, organic milk, fresh eggs and enough vegetables to feed a village of forty!

Even though he was immensely busy every single day, he also took the time to savor life. I remember a moment, sitting with him in the garden under the shade of a small tree, in shared silence.

All he said was, "Let's watch the vegetables grow." There we sat, gazing lovingly at the fecundity that surrounded us. An immense sense of peace filled my heart.

Years later, in his last few hours of life, I recounted this moment to him, letting him know he would live on, in the garden of my heart.

Within each of us is a seed—the seed of what we were born to gift this world.

The desire to contribute is a very important

song. When not heard or heeded, it can leave one awaiting the mercy of Death's kiss.

Some of us know what our gifts are, but more of us are blind to our unique offering, unable to feel its resonant beat in the depths of our hearts.

Most of this is due to the fact that as a young child, our creative impulse to do what was true for our spirit was quickly turned wrong and funneled into a narrow group of options: doctor, lawyer, business man/woman, firefighter and so forth.

It's said that between the ages of four and seven, we express and do what we naturally love, providing a window into our greater gift that has yet to fully emerge.

I remember I was jumping with joy, delighted with life, when suddenly I became aware that my nakedness under my nightgown was odd to the other children, all whom were older than my five year old self.

As we went to sleep on a big mat across the floor, an eleven-year-old boy snuggled up to me and ended up cupping my yoni (vulva) with his small hand. He didn't hurt me or force himself onto me, he just held me.

I lay there frozen, unable to move—not because I was scared, but because a sensation of intense pleasure was spreading through my whole body. In that moment, the neural pathways ignited with conscious awareness of "touch this and wonderful warmth starts to pulse through me."

This is how I discovered I had a very magical place on my body, one that would, reliably, induce the most fantastic sensations. This is how I knew without a doubt, in my five-year-old mind, that my girlfriends had to know about this!

I found myself in the basement of my best friend's house with a small group of my girlfriends. I was showing them the magical place I'd discovered and they were feeling for themselves, with their own bodies, if it was magical for them too.

The fun ended very abruptly, when my best friend's older sister found us. She grabbed me by the hair and dragged me up the stairs to throw me out of her house, all the while calling me "the devil's spawn" and promising me I'd never see any of my friends again.

I remember feeling confused by her anger and absolutely certain about my knowledge—

she must not know about this amazing spot, because if she did she wouldn't be so angry.

So began my career, at the ripe old age of five, sharing love and delight in our beautiful female body and her amazing capacity for pleasure.

I was only five then, but I knew I was right to share about my body and its pleasure.

This never went away, my erotic innocence remained intact, even though I was witness to many atrocities on the Canadian First Nations reservations I grew up on. Perhaps it was the witnessing of women's pain—along with the blessing of being a woman and having a female body—that kindled such a deep spark within, to invite them to remember their sexual sovereignty.

All I know, even now, is there is something bigger than me that pulls me forward, informs me, moves me and blesses me with wisdom beyond my years.

It's my own unique song of desire for contribution.

Our Own Offering

"When we contribute, we connect with the world. When we make a difference, we create meaning for our lives. Contribution goes beyond the self. In this way we connect with the world and hence expand our sense of identity."

ChangingMinds.org

Our contribution doesn't need to be fancy, or to make us a lot of money. Our contribution is our own offering to life and offering it is enough.

Anything less is a hijacked desire of contribution.

Caroline Myss, author of Defy Gratvity, often speaks about the "cruise ship of spirituality," where we believe we are destined to live a glamorous, wealthy, famous life. Yet, she also shares that it's in the simple jobs that the greatest spiritual work can happen. Take, for example, the local mechanic, who just does his job, yet everyone knows him and likes to be around him, because just being in his presence feels both warm and inspiring

That is our life's work: to express shamelessly the gifts we were born with.

If I had done what my parents had wanted me to do, I would have been a doctor or a lawyer. I even considered these things—not because of passion, but because I believed my parents knew better. Sound familiar?

The only person who is an expert on us is ourselves.

Without expressing the song of our inborn gift, we always feel incomplete, as though there is something missing in our world and there is.

"Profound joy of the heart is like a magnet that indicates the path of life."

Mother Theresa

The desire to contribute is such an enlivening song; if it grows too quiet we may actually die. We can see this in older people who no longer feel seen or able to contribute as they did: somehow they appear to diminish in size and potency.

Chapter 9

Knowing Our Desire Song

Well, I always know what I want. And when you know what you want—you go toward it. Sometimes you go very fast, and sometimes only an inch a year. Perhaps you feel happier when you go fast. I don't know. I've forgotten the difference long ago, because it really doesn't matter, so long as you move.

Ayn Rand

It was a stuffy summer day, and for some reason I got it in my head to join a short course in exploring career options. They had us fill out those silly tests where you use a pencil and fill in the little circles that indicated our answers.

When we returned the following week, they announced to each of us what we'd be best suited for. I was told that I should go into science and mathematics. Yes. Dry, boring, and certainly not inspiring. In fact, accounting was even mentioned!

I remember leaving class and crumpling up my results, feeling like maybe I was just too young to worry about a decision that would affect me for the rest of my life.

That very night, I took out my telescope and dreamed about faraway space travel and life in other galaxies. That seemed much more reasonable than accounting.

Desire is a symphony. At times we may be more aware of one song than another, like being more aware of a particular instrument in the orchestra.

Desire is pulling us into who we really are. Desire has a strong imperative—it points to fulfillment and we get to remember the simple truth: *fulfillment is a moment-to-moment realization of how deeply alive we are right now.*

Yet, in a world of incessant to-do lists—the attempt to fulfill hijacked desires—we get the opposite. We use up our own juice in pursuit of fulfillment, which is predetermined by external, unbendable influences.

Therefore, we never know true fulfillment. We are only temporarily filled, and we wonder what all the hype was about, since we feel emptier, shallower, and more desperate than ever before.

Desire is our daemon—the genius of our own essence of fulfillment—of our wholeness, our holiness. Desire isn't something we chose: she chose us in the moment our parents surrendered to the song of creation.

Desire is pure: her intent is to bring you, over and over and over again, back into the state Buddha describes as nirvana, even though nirvana is described as being free from desire.

However, even if all of our great influencers left breadcrumbs about fulfillment for us, our conditioning makes us deaf to their wisdom on fulfillment and the mystery of life. We cannot believe it's that simple: we assume this wisdom must only be for the great saints, who devoted their entire life to self-realization. Or we believe it's only for those who are extremely wealthy and have everything at their fingertips.

But it's not.

The lens of our consensual reality mars this truth.

There is no one in particular to blame—we are all born full of pure, creative potential. We all immediately absorbed the virus offered to us by all who came into our world. We participate in inertia and blindness willingly because we know no other way.

Our desire, because she never goes away or turns off—she cannot—is hijacked. We are conditioned to believe and to be moved by desires that are not genuine to our nature, but rather the ones promoted by a massive machine of industry, government, and religion.

How can we know our true Desire song? Maybe we don't: maybe we still sing the phony songs we've known our whole life.

We all sing the phony songs and we sing them with passion. In time, we feel more and more jaded and empty, only halfheartedly singing or murmuring, more out of habit than out of joy.

Living a Switched-On Life

Therefore, if socialized desire is everywhere and is the cause of much of our ill health, neurosis, and dissatisfaction, then what can we do to change it?

Nothing.

There is nothing to do.

To engage with these socialized constructs at all is to partake in them, even when we believe we are rebelling and choosing to "change" them.

Rather, the solution is quite simple.

We must remember our own pure desire—while simultaneously shedding all of our ideas about desire—and enter into a new relationship with her.

For fun, a friend of mine decided to do an astrology reading for me. I had my suspicions, but she was so excited about sharing her discovery with me.

"You're going to teach about sexuality."

I promptly gave her the finger, picked up my purse, and walked out of her house, absolutely horrified.

I was fuming, how dare she suggest such stupidity? I mean, sex is fun to have, but to make a career out of it? You either have to be a doctor or some wacky New Age person wearing white gowns and "Om-ing"—neither of which appealed to me.

Yet, a few years later, I found myself teaching about sexuality—but in my version, with grounded, clear, embodied integrity. In fact, empowering women around their sexual sovereignty has become my life's work.

Once freed of influences—not because they disappear, but because we change where we put our focus—we are infused with curiosity, vulnerability, and openness.

It takes courage to step out of the powerful plowing of consensual reality. Yet, once we are out, we can see more clearly and can learn again to be innocent, to be simple, and to experience the profound magic that resides in each arising moment.

Take this very moment—we'll never live it again. The poignancy of life becomes an ally, keeping us perpetually aligned with our own true north, our own compass set to the magnetic current our of our own uniqueness.

This is how we can live a switched-on life, it's actually the choiceless choice as we are designed to function this way.

"There is never a single "right way" to do something; Optimal Living is about finding the "best way" for you. It is a personal choice. You decide on the intensity of any changes. You audit the different areas of your life to decide what is working, what needs improvement, and what can stay the same."

Ethan Thane

Yet, even though we are all imbued with the same daemon, the same genius, most of us primarily exist as switched-off beings: numb, addicted, neurotic, desperate, empty, and alone.

Even those of us who claim to be switched-on, actually have only had a moment here and there, where life suddenly animates us—and the rest of the time we're still beggars pleading for the return to bliss. So we use sugar, social media, drama, sex, work, alcohol, and drugs—anything to take us back to that momentary dopamine high.

Still others of us believe—we've convinced ourselves—that we've never felt alive and good. That our lives have been a sequence of tragedies, leaving us comfortable with our version of misery and yet, we still secretly yearn.

We all yearn.

Yearning is how desire whispers to us, true desire never abandons us. She cannot, her sole purpose is to enliven us, and so she does, even if we can only hear the distorted version of her call.

It's curious how we've demonized the very thing—our desire—that can rectify the scales, which can transform despair and depressive boredom into resilient, permeating peace.

The moon was full that summer's eve and the Mediterranean Sea calmer than a lake. We walked in silence toward the water's edge, choosing to sit on a thick bed of soft, sun-dried seaweed.

Held in this stillness, I suddenly became aware I was truly ONE with everything. My heart was so light, so free, and so pure, I finally understood what the ancient saints spoke of: how inner peace—is the most extraordinary experience. Once felt, we are forever changed, for-

ever called back to return to this pristine state of tranquility.

I looked over at my husband and saw him smiling at me; he knew. It felt magnificent to be met and seen in the profundity of this moment.

The Peace of Surrender

To taste inner peace is to know nothing else is even remotely worthy of pursuit. Unlike commonly assumed, peace isn't bland or flaccid or timid. Peace is the all-pervasive state of being that has come to reside fully in the allness of life.

Peace is being porous, touched, inflamed, and engaged. Peace is the note in the symphony that unites all the songs. Peace is the hidden thread that is woven throughout the fabric of life.

Peace—deep, unmoving, profound aliveness, the sensation of wholeness, holiness, completeness, and oneness—is not just for a select few. It belongs to each of us, but the misalignment with our nature prevents us from tasting peace, makes us mistrust our desire.

For far too long we have struggled to attain the promise of fulfillment held within socialized desires. We give our lives to these hijacked songs and we never once question their validity. Desperation and suffering are the results of our pursuit of fulfillment.

Desire isn't reserved only for the privileged: it's the birthright of all who are born into this life. The poor also catch glimpses of their true desires, moments of profound peace amidst their own tumultuous journey.

Desire lives in all of us, for the good, the bad, the beautiful, and the ugly. If we exist, we are imbued with the daemon of desire.

Our journey, therefore, isn't to make our desire more important than another's, or to claim the righteousness of our desire. Our journey is to recognize the voice of our own soul's calling and to make that our true North Star, our magnetic north—so we can always orient ourselves toward that which is already moving toward us.

"Researchers investigating happiness have found the following factors enhance a person's wellbeing: a happy intimate relationship with a partner, a network of close friends, enjoyable and fulfilling career, enough money, regular exercise, nutritional diet, sufficient sleep, spiritual or religious beliefs, fun hobbies and leisure pursuits, healthy self-esteem, optimistic outlook, realistic and achievable goals, sense of purpose and meaning, a sense of belonging, the ability to adapt to change, and living in a fair and democratic society."

Australian Bureau of Statistics

Our collective journey is to acknowledge our hijacked desires and to simply turn our attention back to our deeper song. Back to the deep, resonant fulfillment that arises when we are aligned with life.

For this, we must be willing to stand in our sovereignty, especially when others believe they cannot. Sovereignty, although a human birthright must be claimed, honed, and lived. It's our privilege, our gift.

This means unplugging from consensual reality and risk entering the realm of creating, moment to moment, a new reality: our real life. It means letting go of being a proud victim, of being a numb zombie, of being directed by the will of others rather than our own prime directive.

> *"What was really needed was a fundamental change in our attitude toward life. We had to learn ourselves and, furthermore, we had to teach the despairing men, that it did not really matter what we expected from life, but rather what life expected from us."*
>
> ***Dr. Frankl***

It can be disorienting when we shift into allowing our real life to take the place of the false illusions we once called reality. It can feel frightening, because certainty is something sweetly familiar, something we can control.

This is a little like a seed being terrified of its impending transformation, fearing annihilation. Yes, the seed as a seed shall cease to exist in the form of a seed—but she will come to embody her true potential: the giant oak, the humpback whale, the juicy peach, and the creative human. All of which miraculously contains...more seeds!

In our conditioning, in our terror of aligning with our daemon, we force ourselves to remain a seed, without realizing our deepest calling is to surrender to and become the fullness of who we really are.

Surrender is terrifying for most of us, surrender implies defeat, weakness, losing. But these are false premises. True surrender isn't to a person or thing, it's to life itself.

When we can relax, allow and experience both the law of time (all things have their time to come into fruition) and the law of spaciousness (all beings require a particular degree of space to function fully), we activate our true desire and access fulfillment.

The choice is simple: either we stay comfortable, pouring our essence continuously into false constructs that dry us up and leave a husk of us in their place—or we surrender to our deepest calling.

"I choose to be the predominant creative force in my life."

Robert Fritz

Surrendering is a homecoming, allowing ourselves to finally reside in our sovereignty. Allowing ourselves to embrace our messy imperfections, along with the beauty of our unique soul's song.

The world shall be more gorgeous, more whole, and more alive because of it.

To truly do this, we must constantly confront our conforming tendencies. This doesn't mean smashing windows and spray-painting buildings—but metaphorically, it does.

It means being willing to be sovereign, autonomous, complete unto ourselves. It means no longer seeking approval or perfection, but rather living our moments wholeheartedly.

It means risking the wrath of others, risking everything. Yet, we were dead in that old way of life, comfortable and on the long path of a very slow suicide.

"What's the greater risk? Letting go of what people think—or letting go of how I feel, what I believe, and who I am?"

Dr. Brené Brown

What we'll find, when coming home to ourselves, aligning with our daemon is that our unsung gifts shall emerge and offer themselves in service to the world.

Switched-on people are creators, they contribute. They affect others with their presence, they inspire, touch, move, and bless.

Chapter 10

Daring Our Desires

You only live once, but if you do it right, once is enough.

Mae West

I was in my third week of a total darkness retreat in Thailand. No light, no actual seeing with my physical eyes for three full weeks.

What happens to our body when deprived of light is intriguing to say the least. In the first week, I could not stop sleeping, it was like a lifetime of exhaustion working itself out of my system.

The second week was the most painful; I relived every body trauma I'd ever had, as though it was all happening again! In fact, I was con-

vinced I was dying, that second week. I remember the moment I stopped myself from my panic and thought: Well, no one knows I'm dying, so I'm going to die alone. Is this how I want to spend my last moments? Freaking out? Then I let myself completely relax...and I did not die.

However, it was the third week that was the most spectacular, my consciousness remained awake 24/7. Although my body slept for maybe three to four hours a day, I was awake and aware during this time. During this extremely lucid period, I became in touch with what is called our "spiritual hormones," where we start to experience super-consciousness and to be able to see through the small window of our habitual lives.

It was in those moments, when I was seeing the cosmos and experiencing visuals not unlike those described in DMT journeys, that I tapped into a powerful knowing: I had to truly dive into whatever my essence was calling me toward because life in its normal day-to-day routine would never, ever push me toward these lofty dreams.

There is an element, which, throughout time, has enabled our species to survive and evolve. This element is crucial to transforming the inertia of our conforming tendencies. It awakens our original curiosity and inspires us into action: Daring.

Being daring is essential if we want to live in accordance with our true north, our desire. It's crucial for shifting out of the humdrum and breaking us free from our habitual, less-than-fully-alive life.

Sometimes, it's the little things that dare us the most: getting out of bed after a long sleepless night, saying goodbye to a toxic relationship, or leaving an unfulfilling job.

Being daring is the only way to forge through the inertia of our conditioning. It's our ally because living a fully expressed life requires daring: daring to be who we really are, daring to speak our truth and go for our dreams the real ones, not the ones we've adopted from our culture.

We must dare.

Not daring means we never honor our uniqueness, our soul-song is singularly our own, a magnificent and vital part of the entire symphony of life.

Why do we succumb to our domestication

and a predetermined version of what someone else thinks the "norm" should be?

In nature, everything belongs and has its rightful place. Unique, yet connected. So why do humans believe the monotone, the "requirements of belonging" have any value for us?

Because we don't know any better.

It's the beauty of domestication: once we've adopted it, we continue to self-maintain it!

Self-domestication is the act of accepting ourselves on the condition that we live up to the ideals we have adopted from others in the Dream of the Planet, without ever considering if those ideals are what we truly want.

Don Miguel Ruiz

The Hand Brake of Fear

Fear numbs our human spirit, dampens our will, and puts out the fire of passion.

To wake up enthused, to live our days enthused, to eat and drink enthused, to relate enthused, to partake in any human activity enthused is to live, as the ancient Greeks would say, with *entheos* (meaning "divinely inspired, possessed by a god.)"

This isn't random or just for others: this is how we all could be if we weren't beaten down by fear—the fear of not belonging, of not being good enough, capable enough, or worthy enough. These are learned wounds, wounds that, if indulged, set us on a path of confusion.

On one hand, our natural impulse is toward desire, toward our soul's fulfillment. On the other hand, we yank on the brake of fear, only allowing ourselves to go for what has already been set in motion through social conditioning.

When desire becomes demonic, it erodes us, leaving us empty-handed and jaded, unwilling to allow ourselves to dream, because going for our dreams is either impossible or unfulfilling.

Fulfillment calls us to itself, for its own sake.

Desire Is Our Ally

However, desire becomes our daemon—our trustworthy ally—when we allow ourselves to dive into our deepest yearning and follow it.

Now, understand, desire and fulfillment care not for right/wrong, good/bad: they are invested in you living your most expressed life and that's it.

As we allow ourselves to acknowledge our conditioning and turn our attention to what we love, we must call on our daring nature to assist us with following through.

I worked in a warehouse with no windows and fluorescent lighting, filled with dust. I was running a gourmet seed company for a friend and my job was to triple-clean bird seeds before packaging them.

My shifts started as early as five a.m. in the worst part of downtown Vancouver, with prostitutes and heroine junkies in the streets at all hours of the day and night.

I remember the day I lost it, it was out of character for me to make a fuss: I was normally very calm, even in stressful situations.

Not that day, that day I cracked into a thousand messy pieces. I'm not sure what triggered it.

I angrily kicked one of the boxes out of my way and it felt so good, I did it again and again and again, each kick and punch more powerful, more rewarding than the last. Mix in my screams of frustration and we had a full-on temper tantrum.

I felt calm afterward. A friend's recent words echoed in my heart: "You are not stuck! I've always known you to create. Just create again."

And create I did, I left that job, losing my friendship with the owner, and ended up outdoors as a "bunker babe"—the person who rakes all the sand pits—at a prestigious golf course, making twice the pay (a full $15/hour) and breathing fresh, clean air.

However, I realized this was just me replacing one fear with another lame excuse. It wasn't real daring, as I had yet to heed the deeper yearning in my heart, to open my own private massage practice.

As luck would have it, I got laid off. The debilitating anxiety attacks started that same day.

If you've never suffered from an anxiety attack, it feels like you're dying. Your world closes in on you, you can't breathe, and your heart feels like it's about to race to a full stop.

Little did I know, this was the merciless calling of my contribution to life.

Six months in, I found myself on my knees, whispering to God, "Fine. I'll do my life's work... BUT YOU MUST TAKE CARE OF ME FINANCIALLY! I won't do this poor." I had not yet started to look for work, but did know that my dream job would involve doing massage. And miraculously, the very next day, a call came offering me my "dream" job: working only one week a month at five times the pay ($75/hour), being flown to and from a private billionaire's island resort in a private water plane!

The tips were EPIC! Plus, I was free to build up my own budding massage business. This launched me into living my true desire.

I no longer do massage for a living, but I still very much live the life of my dreams. Has it been easy? Not always. Has it been worth the uncertainty and the insecurity of not knowing what was coming next? Yes, 300 percent.

The aching desire we feel right now—our true desire, our deeper calling—is evolutionary. It only reveals itself through the next obvious step. All we need to do is dare to take it.

I've done many things since that day on my knees, always "daring greatly" as Dr. Brené Brown likes to say, daring into my leading edge. It always feels intense, like: "Wow?! Really?!! This?!?! Can I possibly go for this?!" The answer is always a resounding *"YES!"*

I've been married three times. The first was to the sum of all of my hijacked desires on romance. It lasted for one month before it was annulled. The second was for the curiosity of love and the contract of gaining a green card, which allowed me to live on the beautiful island of Maui for a decade. It ended with him having an affair. The third marriage—well, we met in 2007 and became lovers/partners in 2009 and to this day my heart sings with delight at the dynamic and evolutionary depth of this exquisite relationship.

Daring to live in accordance with our true desires isn't a cookie-cutter experience. There is no manual for a life well lived, only the daily enthusiasm of living it.

We take our life for granted, thinking it will always be there, that the same people will be there forever and we'll relax into a predictable routine—and perhaps, for a few of us, this is true. But for most of us, routine, the known, certainty itself can be like a form of suicide, and a slow one at that.

If we were able to know the precise unfolding of our lives, in hope of eradicating our fears of the unknown, we'd most likely not want to live it—since we'd already know exactly what to expect and how everything would turn out. Is that a life worth living? Hardly.

Instead, let's consider the unknown, the mystery, as an exceptional blessing. We get to create it! We get to make it all up!! We get, at the end of our life, to look back and say with satisfaction and certainty, "I did it. I lived as fully as I could." Our last breath could feel like the ultimate punctuation to a regret-free life.

Regret-Free Living

Most of us already have regrets. Regrets are our own knowing that our true Desire showed up and we turned away from it, opting instead to stay cozy, rather than to lean into the wildness of the edge of our own mystery.

Regrets suck and they burden our hearts.

I still remember this moment like it was yesterday, so strong is the power of regret.

I was at the Baltimore bus station, heading to West Virginia, when I saw him sitting there, across the station, looking my way. Our eyes locked and I instantly felt a strong magnetism, a deep desire to connect.

Instead of going right over, I just sat there, tortured by the yearning of my entire body. When I finally decided to go and say hello, a massive crowd filed out of a bus and swarmed the space between us. By the time the crowd cleared, he was gone and my heart was suddenly heavy with a sensation that would stay with me all week.

It was so awful that I finally decided I would always, from there on, move toward any strong calling, simply so I could avoid collecting any more weighted regrets.

As life has a great sense of humor, it was only a week later, at the same bus station—now wait-

ing to return to NYC—my opportunity arrived.

He was in front of me in the line, and I simply leaned into the amazing heart calling and ended up having an epic adventure with a man that would become a good friend and sweet lover.

"Our choices determine the destiny of the world. By making a choice, you alter the structure of reality."

Jordan B. Peterson

I knew I could not and would not continue to collect regrets like pearls on a heavy necklace. I knew the only way to be regret-free was to say YES to my soul-song, especially if it had me catching my breath in anticipation.

With my third husband, when we first got together, there was a grey zone of "closure" between him and his ex. At times, it felt as if there was too much of her in our newly forming life.

One afternoon, I sat quietly with my hands resting on my heart and I asked myself, "What would you love?"

My clear answer:"I'd love to experience his full, devotional love." I let myself hear that and receive that desire. I then contemplated how it would feel if my heart's desire were true.

In that moment, I experienced a deep fulfillment, a sensation of living truth, even though my current situation did not yet reflect this. I felt the truth of his deep, unwavering love, and then I let it go, having tasted the fruition of my desire in its full form.

Wouldn't you know—soon after, he called me and professed his newly made choice to claim me as his own. To this day, his devotion has emerged more and more. What is most amazing is that it feels exactly like it did on that initial afternoon when I meditated on my heart's desire.

This is not meant to paint the image of perfect relating. Humans are naturally very messy and my husband and I are not exempt from this. Yet, messiness and all, our love continues to evolve and thrive.

"Knowing how you actually want to feel is the most potent form of clarity that you can have."

Danielle LaPorte

Chapter 11

Tension is Creative

The starting point of all achievement is desire.

Napoleon Hill

I was very fond of my new lip-gloss and wanted my friend to smell it, so I said to her, "Smell my lips."

She had cinnamon sprinkles on her little nose and the kind of mouth I'd describe as extremely kissable. She was tall, a little chubby in a sexy sort of way, and knew her way around the garden like no one's business.

She seemed a little startled by my request, perhaps because in her lesbian world, one did not make such overt moves. Nevertheless, she leaned in to take a long sniff of my glistening lips.

In that moment, an electric spark arched between our mouths and startled both of us. I felt a powerful urge to kiss her, even though I had a boyfriend and she had clearly let me know she had a girlfriend.

I didn't kiss her, but instead grew to enjoy a certain zing-like tension that would rise whenever she came close to me. I was incredibly surprised, since I hadn't been into women before. Relishing in our ever-growing sexual tension, I was able to relax and enjoy the lively effect of her presence.

With desire, inevitably comes tension, and tension is something most of us try to relieve as soon as the smallest hint of it arises. But if we are too quick to resolve our tension, then we end up dissatisfied and flat-lined.

In some—most, actually—tension is necessary for functioning.

What allows an arch bridge to span greater distances than a beam bridge, or a suspension bridge to stretch over a distance seven times that of an arch bridge? The answer lies in how each bridge type deals with the important forces of compression and tension.

Robert Lamb & Michael Morrissey

Leaning Into Tension

For a lot of us, the idea of "leaning into tension"—feeling it, yet not attempting to resolve it instantly—isn't inspiring. On the contrary, it can be annoying, frustrating, and at times, exasperating.

In a culture where instant gratification is the prioritized, tension is merely an indication to consume more, and more quickly.

Let's take sexual tension as an example, there is power, a magical space between two (or more) people, when Ero's potential arises, but isn't acted upon. Remember your first kiss? The electricity between your mouth and the other persons? There's intensity there, there is LIFE there. To kiss too quickly would ruin the moment.

Personally, I often prefer sexual tension to resolution because I've learned to enjoy the voltage that electrifies the air around me. In fact, in many cases, the right decision for me isn't to "resolve" the tension. However, instead of just shutting down and making it wrong, I relax. I relax into the rising arousal and let it touch me deeply, electrifying my every cell.

I know full well it's the tension itself that fulfills me, not its resolution. Being able to sit with tension can save us a lot of drama, as often we are too quick to act and then we regret our choices. Our ability to take a breath, understanding that we do have the capacity to relax into the rising intensity, while remaining aware of all of ourselves, helps us to contribute to making conscious choices we are happy to live with.

This is crucial in responding to the call of our desire. Many of my students have reported that through the practice of my method of the Jade Egg (a psycho-sexual practice of using an egg-shaped piece of real Jade intra-vaginally), they have felt powerful shifts in handling bad habits and tension-resolution patterns.

For example, a woman who suffered from an emotional eating disorder, started to do my method of the Jade Egg practice regularly and noticed that her eating issue transformed itself naturally and gave her the spaciousness to relax in the face of her triggers. In fact, her eating disorder all but disappeared, purely from the act of coming into right relationship with herself and her body.

This has also happened with women who shop or have sex in order to fulfill an emptiness they feel, and who desire to resolve their habit. They too found that their need to react to life shifted and they became more conscious and aware of making true, satisfying choices.

"If your dreams do not scare you, they are not big enough."

Ellen Johnson Sirleaf

Some of our desires will scare us: if they don't, they may be false desires. Remember, we are conditioned to deal with our desires by seeking instant gratification or suffering from frustration and/or disillusionment.

When we align with our soul's calling, sometimes we won't understand *how it will happen*. That's where letting go of the need to know is very helpful. Personally, I have never known what would emerge from my conscious choices—I just knew I was willing to meet it wholeheartedly.

That's life: meeting what emerges with a state of grace, enthusiasm, and wonderment. This is true even in the smallest of moments.

My grandmother had nine children and two miscarriages. She was poor, busy, and I was told, a living angel. To my five-year-old heart she was more of a living goddess. She was always kind, joyous, honest, and willing to do what it took to bring joy into your life.

Near where she lived, there was a park full of junkies and questionable characters, so none of the local kids would play there. Since no one else wanted to take on this task, my grandmother singlehandedly transformed this park into a clean, safe area for kids of all ages to enjoy.

She told my mother we should do all of our tasks, no matter how menial (such as the cleaning of a toilet), with joy in our hearts. This attitude alone was one of the secrets to her powerful and grace-filled life.

We all have an internal compass, one revealing whether we're switched on or switched off. When we operate from a *switched-off* place, no matter what our external circumstances are, we'll never see the beauty in the simple and we'll always be one of the "have-nots"—the ones who never have enough time, money, inspiration, etc. to truly live the life they were given.

No matter our circumstances, when we choose to exist from a *switched-on* state, we can BE with what we are attending to without identifying with it. a It actually doesn't mean anything about us, if we clean toilets or take out the trash or work at an unglamorous job or drive an older car or don't have the latest version of the smart phone. These things have no meaning except the meanings we assign to them.

"The miracle is not that we do this work, but that we are happy to do it."

Mother Teresa

How fully we partake in all our moments is what gives our lives meaning. Do we let the warmth of the spring sun melt us open? Or allow the soft, sultry breeze of a summer's night to caress us? Are we able to really see the stranger who happens to meet our eyes?

These moments are not random—they are our life. Unique. Messy. Human. Beautiful. Fulfillment doesn't have a particular timeline: fulfillment only cares how deeply we live with each breath.

Creative Orientation

Fulfillment is a moment-to-moment gift that we give ourselves when we choose the life of living with our own true north as our guide.

There is wisdom in this orientation, which is known as the *creative orientation* to life. The creative orientation is the capacity to tune into and say YES to our heart's calling or our true desires, while also honestly acknowledging the current reality we find ourselves in at this moment.

CREATIVE ORIENTATION = THE TRUTH OF THIS MOMENT
+ OUR TRUE DESIRES.

It doesn't end there! When we examine what we are currently living, what we yearn for, we find there is often a discrepancy between those two polarities. In the creative orientation, this discrepancy is considered a powerful resource, a source of creative tension.

As you may remember from the previous chapter, holding tension creates more aliveness for us. Creative tension is no different. In fact, in the creative orientation, creative tension is very desirable as it propels us to move toward our true desires.

The capacity to love and hold our creative tension is a skill we are not taught, and one that is weakened through our social conditioning of resolving tension as soon as it arises, especially if the tension is very strong. Yet, we all can become more masterful with this facet of creating.

Our capacity to be daring—along with truth and our true desires—makes up the sacred trinity of our creative orientation to life. Being authentically daring is our ability to say YES to and act in an honest, dedicated, and consistent way toward the actualization of our true desires.

In other words, being daring is both our capacity to hold creative tension and our capacity to take clear, obvious action—do what's obvious, to do right in the moment—toward realizing our deepest calling.

CREATIVE ORIENTATION = TRUTH + TRUE DESIRES + DARING.

The ability to both hold the creative tension between our present-moment and what we desire, coupled with our ability to exercise our will and act in alignment with our true desire, results in the emergence of our daring nature.

Our will isn't something we fully understand, much less revere, in this culture. For most of us, the idea of will is the use of *force* to do something, such as, the idea of willpower. Yet our will, our ability to act, is part of our sovereignty and our capacity to create the life yearning to come through us.

It takes will and guts to live an expressed, fulfilled, and creative life. Anything less results in living someone else's idea of our ideal life.

"In a society that benefits from your self-doubt, liking yourself is a rebellious act."

Shamash Alidina

It's worth mentioning that the demonic aspect of desire surfaces when we attempt to resolve an emerging tension instantly, without thought or spaciousness around whether or not this "choice" is truly conscious. Resolving tension too quickly often leads us further away from fulfillment and aliveness.

The daemonic desire, however, only wants us to experience the full expression of our creative power. We may not know how this desire will fulfill itself and it's not our job to know.

It's simply our job to claim, and to meet whatever arises from it with certainty and daring. No matter what comes, we'll meet it as an enthusiastic and whole being.

As a switched-on human, we have access to far more talent and resources than we've ever been allowed to feel and express.

We were not born to be like everyone else.

"Why fit in when you were born to stand out!"

Dr. Suess

There isn't one single snowflake that is identical to another, so why should we succumb to the boring 'cookie-cutter' replica that fashion, media, religion, family, and government want to impose on us?

Our need to belong, to conform, will rise over and over again, until we make friends with it and dare to choose to realize our desires, enjoying the immense creative power that comes from this tension.

Chapter 12

When Desire Disappears

Desire begins in the mind.

Paola Franco, Dangerous Beauty

Why did I agree to four months of celibacy?! Never in my life had I not masturbated, though I had periods of choosing not to be sexually active with others. But not being able to touch myself? That was outrageous!

In fact, the first two weeks of this self-inflicted jail time was horrendous. Not only did I have to go away from my husband, as his proximity was utter torture (for both of us), but a deep, throbbing pain built up in my lower abdomen, so strongly that I had to either press myself into the hard corner of the counter top or get a girlfriend to spank me as hard as she could, while tears of frustration would stream down my face—either of these scenarios would help relieve the building agony in my pelvis.

And then the worst happened.

I lost all life inside of me, the ever-present pulse in my vagina was dead. My body seemed to be withering more and more with each passing day.

It felt worse than death, because I was forced to function in a lifeless state.

Sometimes desire cannot be felt, heard, or even imagined. We've gotten so lost in the stories of our lives that we're not even aware we've become deaf to the very thing we yearn for most: fulfillment.

When desire is quiet, it doesn't mean it's gone. There may be a pause, in relation to sensing our desire. It's as though desire goes deeper within, to source the next nuance of our heart's calling.

If we can relax and trust in this much-needed incubation stage of creating, we'll find that fairly quickly, desire returns with even more fervor than before.

But sometimes, it's not creative liberation that's causing us to feel the lack of desire's visceral calling. Sometimes it's purely because we are so immersed in our own conditioned story that we are numb to our desire's presence.

Do you have a favorite story? One you infuse with your emotional energy and righteousness? We all have such a story. If you feel you don't, don't worry, you're just in denial—none of us are exempt from this story-making and story-telling tendency.

It's the current story of our life and only a few recognize the difference between, when we are story-telling and when we are actually being the creator of our lives.

Our stories are our security blankets. We carry them wherever we go, and pull them out to soothe the agitation we feel when we,

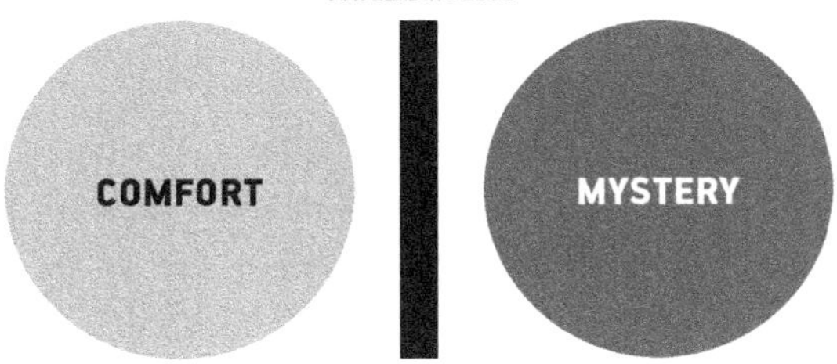

by chance or intent, arrive closer to our own leading edge—the edge where, what is comfortable for us and what is unknown, combine. This isn't just any unknown, but the unknown of our own greatness, our own essential gift in its full realization.

Therefore, these ever-present stories we repeatedly tell ourselves, actually numb us, pulling us away from our own power—our ability to act in the world, our daring nature.

It's scary to contemplate living on our leading edge, because what we know won't be very useful here. It's our mystery, our personal unknown, that holds the answers, the map.

Although, few of us are willing to risk letting go of what we know for the sake of stepping into the unknown.

Letting Go of What We Know

This is where daring comes in handy.

"When we walk to the edge of all the light we have and take a step into the darkness of the unknown, we must believe that one of two things will happen. There will be something solid for us

to stand on or we will be taught to fly."

Patrick Overton

We don't need to assign our faith to a "greater power" outside of us: in fact, faith is an invitation to claim *our own* power, our own limitless creatrix. This is actually what enlivens us.

I remember looking out of my hospital window at all the lucky people walking down the street, oblivious to how precious their life was, absorbed, most likely, in the dramas of their day-to-day life.

I envied their ignorance.

Because I was sitting with the truth that the days were ticking by since the surgeon announced my imminent death.

Yet I knew, somehow, underneath the fear and anger, that I would somehow live, that my time had not yet come to an end. And if that were indeed true, I promised I would make the most of each of my days from this moment forward, never again allowing the pettiness of my own life to dull my reverence of it's actual mystery.

I promised myself I would, when my day did finally arrive, smile in the face of death and say before relaxing into my final surrender: "I did it! I lived, loved, and created as fully as I could in all my moments."

I remember well when an older friend was coming face to face with her mortality. She had a growing urgency to express, to the best of her ability, the fullness of her desire song.

Coming home to ourselves is no small thing. It's not merely a claiming of our individual sovereignty, it's equally a shifting consciousness allowing, that which is true, pure, and inherent within us (our primal genius) to join forces with our soul.

This seemingly simple act of allegiance is more potent and powerful, like the rising of unbridled personal power, confidence and creativity. The full acceptance of ourselves as the true creator of our lives, offering our greatest gifts, means becoming the force of nature we were born to be.

Now imagine a world in which each person truly sheds his or her social cloak and steps forward to live as fully expressed, creative, and contributing individuals.

This new society of genius-infused humans would have the power to change our current world conditions—indeed, the power to create a world that has not yet been dreamed of.

We need everyone's inherent genius to be awake, collaborating with the next evolution of humankind. This emerging expression of our daemon will imbue all facets of our life.

Chapter 13

The Hidden Truth of Desire

The best and most beautiful things
in this world cannot be seen or even
heard, but must be felt with the heart.

Helen Keller

My boyfriend, his best friend, his sister and I were lying in the middle of a quiet street in Winnipeg, laughing uncontrollably at the beauty and ridiculousness of life.

We were witnessing the demise of our domesticated reality as it was turned inside out, revealed in its true form: silly, boring, and full of petty fears.

I still remember the moment we all understood it. The northern lights, dancing their haunting green dance above us seemed to highlight the silent knowing that was passing between us.

In this intangible, irrational, expanded space, our young bodies heard the call of our own true north. We grew reverently silent, as though talking would cause this moment to shatter. As we passed through the eye of the needle, a deeper understanding of our place within the grand symphony of the cosmos emerged.

Desire has been around a lot longer than we have—and much to her amusement, for as long as we've had the capacity to debate, we've been deliberating over desire.

Thousands of arguments and theories for understanding the deeper secrets of desire have emerged from philosopher and scholar alike, but rarely has she been addressed as our daemon.

Maybe it was the desire to impress peers and/or to do well in school, causing emerging insights to become more confusing, rather than liberating to many teens and young adults. Maybe the influence of age-old religions that made our daemon into a demon, striking fear in the hearts of any who dared touch upon their own soul's calling.

Whatever the case, being alienated from our own true north has made it simple for the few to lead the many. When we divert our powerful, creative nature to animate the predetermined vision and desires of the few, we obviously ignore and lose track of our own heart's calling.

In any case, when we seek to understand the nature of life, of Eros, of desire and fulfillment, purely through the lens of our intellect, we can essentially only offer two opinions: 1) what we've already been socialized and indoctrinated into thinking, perceiving, and believing, and 2) what we know of our own living experience of life. Both of which reveal an incomplete story of the mystery of desire.

The Mystery of Desire

Desire has been defined as what "drives us to take action": as what distracts us from what is true, pure, and saintly. Most debates and academic studies attempt to cut desire into digestible, safe, and controllable bits, leaving us no closer to wooing and claiming our own daemon of desire.

In fact, these attempts smell of a couple assumptions: that we are powerless to our desires and that desire is a necessary, yet unholy, part of being human.

Is this true? Is the breaking down of our nature into neuro-chemicals and clever theories bringing us any closer to ourselves? Or is this yet another mechanistic attempt to define the mystery of life?

Perhaps it's the mystics and poets who are closest to the pulse of desire's true nature, sweetly attempting to use words to define that which, in the end, must be tasted and felt personally to be understood.

"Every desire of your body is Holy. Dear one,
Why wait until you are dying to discover that
divine Truth?"

Hafiz

Is desire smiling a crooked smile of amusement at our attempts to buffer her influence through the use of mental constructs?

What matters is that she is our inborn ally.

"[The] power of the Daemon is in the symbolic."

Philosopher's Secret Fire

While words and mental constructs are logical and seemingly trustable and clear, the symbolic—messages we receive faster than words and thoughts—is the language of our intuition. It is said, intuition is the instant knowing that occurs before thoughts and feelings can be imposed upon it.

By allowing ourselves to trust in this aspect of our inherent nature, which has served us long before our alienation from life, we begin to reform our inborn relationship with the mystery of life.

From this porous, diffused, and instantaneous awareness, we access a greater amount of the 400 billion bits of information that flows into our consciousness every single second. It is here we sense the emergence of our own daemon of desire, for she speaks to us in symbols and visceral knowing.

Even though we savvy humans have found ways to objectify desire and have succumbed to the allure of the multitudes of hijacked desires, these powerful imposters have no real say when we align ourselves with our own nature.

"We must have the daring to be nothing but ourselves if we are to know what true power is."

Danielle LaPorte

This is why, when I teach women about their bodies, their sensuality, and their sexuality, I insist they self-define their pleasure, to give it its authentic, sovereign place in their lives.

If I were to fulfill their initial urge to know how it all works—how can I be sexier, more sensual, more orgasmic, and healthier—I would only reinforce the neural pathways of domestication.

Instead, in an oxytocin-infused space of relaxed arousal, each woman is invited to truly inhabit herself, to come into direct relationship with her own daemon of desire.

She was a shadow of what she used to be, small, fragile, and brittle. In fact, I didn't notice her amongst the vibrancy of the rest of the group. Yet, she showed up and she applied herself to all the invitations my weekend provided. And continued to do so for three more months until I returned, once again, to run a follow-up session.

I noticed her instantly: radiant, confident, and fuller somehow. She shared that over the three months she'd practiced, she not only felt younger, she actually rejuvenated her pelvic floor and her sexual health to the point where authentic desire reemerged strongly enough to encourage this gorgeous, seventy-four-year-old woman, to accept and enjoy a relationship with a fifty-two-year-old man.

Desire is ageless, she lives outside of time. False desires cause aging: they are linked to time and energy like insatiable, hungry ghosts.

Desire and Embodied Leadership

As influencers and people who have influence in the lives of others—we must come to recognize the potency of our presence, and always be of service to the sovereignty in others. Putting people in the victim box or leaving them there, only perpetuates powerlessness and the cycle of hopelessness.

Rather, as influencers our sole job is to embody our own living truth, and to trust that it's enough. Through embodied leadership, we remind others that they have the same within them.

By holding the creative tension between how others are now and where they want to be, we empower them to have the same spacious acceptance of their human journey. We empower them to dare into their desires.

Throughout our own journey, our daemon leads us, keeping the spark in our hearts alive. Sometimes the spark is deeply personal and sometimes it's transpersonal: in a way, it's always both. As wisdom of old would say, "As within, so without."

"To be what we are, and to become what we are capable of becoming, is the only end of life."

Robert Louis Stevenson

We must also trust in the daemon within others, respecting each individual's call to create. Through our own embodied action, we must demonstrate how to live within a world of delusion and socialized desires and still be the creatrix of our soul's song.

Here's where definition creates reality.

What are we creating right now? How did we define this very day? This life is ours and ours alone to live. Notice, inertia sneaks into our moments.

Perhaps this is why the ancient oracle of Delphi would insist our first and fundamental lesson was to "Know thyself." Not the clever knowing of learned constructs, but the simple gnosis of who we are beyond all of our adopted definitions.

Back in my twenties, I was a social butterfly, with literally hundreds of friends, all great people I adored and cared for. They came from many different facets of my life: martial arts, belly dancing, aroma-bodywork, qi gong and Tuina, scuba diving, and of course, TV and Film acting.

Just before leaving my "petri-dish" of Vancouver for my heart's-calling of Maui, I threw myself a going away party. I asked everyone to bring a flower that represented their personality as well as an offering that spoke from their hearts.

The bouquet we co-created was spectacular in its diversity of beauty and the evening itself was a profoundly breathtaking talent show! We had no idea what the living talent was, held within this community and we all joyfully received every offer—from opera and violinists, to exotic belly dancing and Bruce Lee-style martial arts feats, to poetry, story, and laughter.

It was gorgeous—the best party I'd ever been to—and it filled my heart far more than just a "good-bye and good-luck," ever could have. It showed me that each of us has a creative genius that is unique and contributes to the beauty of the whole.

It's one thing to cultivate sovereignty for ourselves, and it's another to start to extend that know-how, out to others in our life. A simple way to begin creating the space for others to express their sovereign gifts is through the quality of our listening.

We can choose to listen in such a way where, what is being shared, is unworthy of our attention or is profoundly evocative. Depending on the quality of our listening, the speaker will experience their talk as "bombed" or "best ever." This has been demonstrated experientially.

What this means is who we are and how we show up, influences our experience and those around us. It's the pulse of embodied leadership and each of us are leaders in our own right.

How do we show up? Are we inviting or rigid? Are our expectations of how things should be shaping how things *are*? Lending our enthusiasm and spaciousness enables everyone to thrive (ourselves included).

We can know we are living our true north when the efforts required of us to realize our desire, do not phase us, and we can know we are out of alignment and energizing false desires, when any required effort feels like we are moving mountains.

"Everyone has been made for some particular work, and the desire for that work has been put in every heart."

Rumi

Desire in Action

True Desires will ask everything of us, it's not a free ride down Easy Street. But because fulfillment is a moment-to-moment experience; we can accept the tasks at hand with an unwavering clarity and the satisfaction of doing what it takes.

There's a theory in business that we should be bringing our A game and hiring a team who is each bringing their A game—doing what they love and what they are great at.

But most of us are actually bringing our B game—what we like and are okay at, so long as we don't have to do it for too long—or, worse, our C game—what we hate and suck at.

We can see that if everyone were bringing their unique A game, we'd have more fun and be more effective and productive. This is desire in action, both at work and in the rest of our lives.

Living with our daemon of desire as our ally, has incredible influence on our well being, our capacity to contribute, and our influence in our world.

Living out of touch with her, enmeshed in the web of desires, we burn out, become a burden to those around us, and lose the oomph that comes when we are living as our true selves.

Life is a promise; fulfill it.

Mother Teresa

We can make living in alignment with our desires real at any given moment. What separates true desire from socially mandated desire is simply a choice.

Conclusion

In order to live a fascinating life–one brimming with art, music, intrigue, and romance–you must surround yourself with precisely those things.

Unknown

Desire will never give up on us, even if we give up on her—or, worse, on ourselves.

Desire is the one breathing through us, every breath a yearning of our lungs to know and be connected with life; Desire keeps our hearts beating, a yearning of our body to meet life, whether we are asleep, sick, rocking it out, or resting in quietude.

Desire reminds our belly to digest and our kidneys to filter. Desire can be felt in the breeze, the rain, and the dewdrops sparkling in the grass.

Desire is the heart, the breath, and the impulse for life to keep blossoming.

Desire sings us all into being and keeps us animated throughout our journey. She is the voice of our true north, calling us to live a rich and fulfilling life—to be fulfilled.

Desire is not meant to be philosophized or theorized, but to be felt in the gaps between our thoughts. Desire cares not for your status or baubles, she cares only for one thing: *that your song is sung to its completion*. Each note is brought to fruition and loved for its singularity within the greater symphony.

Desire never abandons us, no matter what we believe or decide.

Desire is you and you are desire.

You can never be separate, because you are one. You were born of desire and shall return to her with your last breath.

Desire is the daemon translating our soul's calling to our human hearts, in simple and profoundly moving ways. In ways that speak not in words, but in the symbolic language of our intuitive and felt nature—the visceral whispering of our trillion cells. Can you hear them? Vibrating, pulsating, radiating your heart-song. This is the only song they know, the song of you and your achingly beautiful uniqueness.

Every fiber of your existence is attuned to your daemon, she is the grand conductor of your personal symphony.

Woo her, adore her and pay attention to her. She imbues your life with magic and makes the impossible plausible.

Her greatest gift is to seduce you into knowing your own fulfillment—not as a bargaining chip, but as your moment-to-moment realization.

The best part? There is no right or wrong way to be with your desire. There is only the choice to do so. How beautiful our human journey is, so exquisitely mysterious and all that's needed is to receive it to the best of our current abilities.

For this, I am grateful.

I'm equally grateful for you, for having taken the time to go on this adventure into desire with me. For this, I am filled with humbled awe.

Together, we are part of this mystery and together we weave the tapestry of life with our uniqueness and spunk.

To our yearning, may she speak in her achingly sweet voice and may we be constantly enamored with her song.

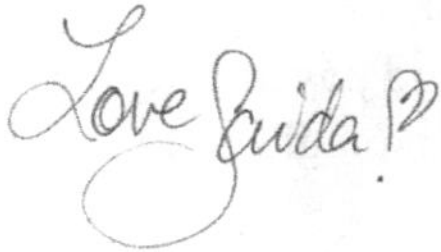

Desire Manifesto

Desire gets a bad rap.

Like the presence of Mae West on the tip of our consciousness.

It's alluring, enlivening, and threatening.

But desire's trial doesn't end here.

Not only does it affect the non-believer, it horrifies and terrifies believers of many great religions.

Still, there is something gorgeous about desire:

It never really goes away.

It shows up every spring in the newly unfurling green and the mating songs that create a symphony of life.

It wakes up the world.

It wakes us up.

Fundamentally, desire is life.

When denied, we shut down. The world becomes a continual landscape of gray, filled with the eerie ring of the monotone.

Nothing tastes, nothing smells, and nothing feels... We are numb.

We are proof that zombies do walk this Earth.

However, when desire, even after years of denial, is given a breath, a quickening happens.

A pulse, a rhythm linked to something older than our "baubles" and "religion," older even than our species.

Within each of us is a prime directive, an encoded force that we cannot measure, yet know of, because without it there is no life.

To be willing to unfetter our desire is to say, "YES" to life, and with that, we are switched on, lit up, ignited, and our unborn gifts finally have the space to emerge.

It's the fulfillment of desire that is the fulfillment of our destiny, our dharma, and our raison d'être.

The choice to truly hear and align ourselves with desire is the choice of aligning our inner compass with true north.

Like all adventures, nothing is ever as it seems. There are trials and initiations that all appear at every new curve in the road. The greatest of these is our human impulse to conform—ensuring our survival through our need to belong.

Now, more than ever, as our very evolution rests in our own hands, we face perhaps our greatest adversary: *a mass illusion of what it means to be fully alive, conscious, creative and contributing human beings.*

And this is where desire kicks in.

Dare your desire...

Acknowledgments

My daemon who ignited and fanned the flame of this little book, first whispering the possibility in 2013, and then, literally leading me to both Africa and Costa Rica as fertile ground for the ideas held within these pages.

My team, for being aligned to my vision and gifting me your greatness in service to touching the lives of women all over the globe, you free me up to do what I do best.

My community, for being the 'early-adopters' to my ideas, for your sovereignty, your heart, and your consistent questions and celebration.

My editors & publisher, for your words of encouragement, your brilliance, and your willingness to co-create with me, receiving my unusual requests with respect and support.

My coaches, for the loving bitch-slaps and ass-kicking that up-leveled my leadership and the way in which I show up in the world.

My close friends, you know who you are, thank you for your ceaseless devotion to showing up with a wide open heart and for 'having my back' and cheerleading me through this creative adventure.

My parents, for not only creating me, but also for inspiring me throughout my life to 'dream and become that which I dream myself to be' and for always believing in me.

My beloved, for the depth of your every touch, for the healing salve of your generous kisses, and for your deep presence cracking me open to greater and greater levels of beauty, love and adventure.